EMERGENCY NURSING

5-Tier
Triage Protocols

EMERGENCY NURSING

5-Tier Triage Protocols

Julie K. Briggs, RN, BSN, MHA
Manager Emergency Services
Providence St. Vincent Medical Center
Portland, Oregon

Valerie G. A. Grossman, RN, BSN, CEN
Senior Nurse Counselor
Via Health: Call Center
Rochester, New York

◆ LIPPINCOTT WILLIAMS & WILKINS
A **Wolters Kluwer** Company
Philadelphia • Baltimore • New York • London
Buenos Aires • Hong Kong • Sydney • Tokyo

Acquisitions Editor: Judy McCann
Editorial Assistant: Katherine Rothwell
Project Manager: Cynthia Rudy
Senior Production Manager: Helen Ewan
Senior Managing Editor / Production: Erika Kors
Design Coordinator: Joan Wendt
Senior Manufacturing Manager: William Alberti
Production Services / Compositor: TechBooks
Printer: R. R. Donnelley–Crawfordsville

9 8 7 6 5 4 3 2 1

Library of Congress Cataloging-in-Publication Data

Briggs, Julie K.
   Emergency nursing : 5-tier triage protocols / Julie K. Briggs, Valerie G. A. Grossman.
      p. ; cm.
   Includes bibliographical references and index.
   ISBN 1-58255-371-8 (alk. paper)
  1. Emergency nursing--Handbooks, manuals, etc. 2. Triage (Medicine)--Handbooks, manuals, etc. I. Grossman, Valerie G. A.
II. Title.

   [DNLM: 1. Triage—methods—Handbooks. 2. Emergencies—nursing—Handbooks. 3. Emergency Service, Hospital—
Handbooks.
WY 49 B854e 2006]
RT120.E4B745 2006
610.73'6—dc22
                                                                                                    2005015208

Care has been taken to confirm the accuracy of the information presented and to describe generally accepted practices. However, the authors, editors, and publisher are not responsible for errors or omissions or for any consequences from application of the information in this book and make no warranty, express or implied, with respect to the content of the publication.

The authors, editors, and publisher have exerted every effort to ensure that drug selection and dosage set forth in this text are in accordance with the current recommendations and practice at the time of publication. However, in view of ongoing research, changes in government regulations, and the constant flow of information relating to drug therapy and drug reactions, the reader is urged to check the package insert for each drug for any change in indications and dosage and for added warnings and precautions. This is particularly important when the recommended agent is a new or infrequently employed drug.

Some drugs and medical devices presented in this publication have Food and Drug Administration (FDA) clearance for limited use in restricted research settings. It is the responsibility of the health care provider to ascertain the FDA status of each drug or device planned for use in his or her clinical practice.

LWW.com

Contributor and Reviewers

Contributor

Theresa Tavernero, RN, BSN, CEN, MHA
Nurse Consultant
Tacoma, Washington

Reviewers

Marge Bentler, RN, BSN, CEN
Emergency Department
Good Samaritan Hospital
Puyallup, Washington

Michael Brook, MD, FACEP
Emergency Medicine
Good Samaritan Hospital
Puyallup, Washington
Clinical Assistant Professor of Medicine
University of Washington Medical Center
Seattle, Washington

Bret Lambert, MD, FACEP
Emergency Medicine
Good Samaritan Hospital
Puyallup, Washington
Clinical Assistant Professor of Medicine
University of Washington Medical Center
Seattle, Washington

Theresa Tavernero, RN, BSN, CEN, MHA
Nurse Consultant
Tacoma, Washington

Preface

The Need for 5-Level Triage Protocols

Today, most emergency departments in the United States, Canada, United Kingdom, Australia, and New Zealand use some type of triage acuity system to determine how quickly a patient needs to be seen and who can safely wait until rooms or resources are available to provide the necessary care. While the most common system has been the 3-tier system that rates patients as Emergent, Urgent, or Non-Urgent, the 5-tier triage system is rapidly gaining momentum as the system of choice. Studies have shown that hospitals using a 5-tier system have reported greater consistency and accuracy in triage decisions. In 2002, the Emergency Nurses Association adopted a resolution promoting 5-level triage in the United States.

In today's rapidly changing health care environment, an efficient emergency department is critical to providing appropriate care at the appropriate time in the appropriate setting. A 5-level triage system helps to ensure that patients are not over-triaged, which depletes scarce resources that may be needed for a patient requiring immediate intervention, or under-triaged, which puts the patient at risk for deterioration while waiting to be seen. *Emergency Nursing: 5-Level Triage Protocols* will assist the triage nurse to function in a more consistent, reliable, and safe manner. The five levels are Resuscitation, Emergent, Urgent, Semi-Urgent, and Non-Urgent, and they are based on patient acuity, severity of symptoms, the degree of risk for deterioration while waiting, and the need for additional resources. In the protocols, ascending levels of urgency are indicated by bolder headings and darker red icons and shading.

This protocol manual can help to achieve the following goals:

- Provide consistency in triage decisions among different nurses
- Utilize healthcare resources in the most appropriate manner
- Set minimum expectations for triage decisions
- Guide the nurse in asking the right questions
- Assist the nurse in determining how soon the patient needs to be seen
- Remind the nurse of interventions to consider
- Serve as a reference for experienced nurses
- Aid the less-experienced nurse in conducting the triage assessment
- Serve as a training tool in orientation

Protocol Components

Each protocol has been developed to ensure accuracy and consistency among the different protocols. Each protocol includes the following:

Title: Protocols are arranged alphabetically and are symptom-based. There are a few diagnosis-based protocols, such as diabetic problems or asthma, which are based on a known diagnosis or past history.

Key Questions: These questions prompt the nurse to routinely ask for baseline and background information. To assist the nurse in meeting JCAHO and regulatory agency requirements, a prompt to ask about the pain scale and measure vital signs is included in the Key Questions of all the protocols. The pain scale used is to be determined by each facility. Other key questions are protocol-specific and prompt the nurse to measure oxygen saturation or ask about the mechanism of injury or tetanus immunization status.

Acuity Level/Assessment and Nursing Considerations: The assessment is categorized from Level 1 through Level 5, with the most severe and life-threatening symptoms listed first in Level 1.

Level 1—Resuscitation: This category is critical and the patient's condition is life-threatening if not managed immediately. In assigning this acuity, the nurse should consider that the patient's condition could quickly deteriorate and will require multiple staff at the bedside, mobilization of the resuscitation team, and many resources.

Level 2—Emergent: This category is high risk for a patient waiting for treatment. The patient's condition could deteriorate rapidly if treatment is delayed. In assigning this acuity, the nurse should consider that the patient will require multiple diagnostic studies or procedures, frequent consultation with the physician, and continuous monitoring.

Level 3—Urgent: This category is moderate risk for a patient waiting to be seen. The patient's condition is stable, but treatment should be provided as soon as possible to relieve distress and pain. Each facility should determine acceptable waiting times if a room is not immediately available. In assigning this acuity, the nurse should consider that the patient may need multiple diagnostic studies or procedures and should be monitored for changes in condition while waiting.

Level 4—Semi-Urgent: This category is low risk for deterioration while the patient is waiting. Symptoms are less severe and the patient can safely wait for treatment. Each facility should determine acceptable waiting times if a room is not immediately available. In assigning this acuity, the nurse should consider that the patient may need a simple diagnostic study or procedure. Patients should be reassessed while waiting, per facility protocol. To enhance customer service, the nurse should offer comfort measures.

Level 5—Non-Urgent: This category is a lower risk for further deterioration while the patient is waiting. Generally, this category of patient could be seen in a lower acuity treatment area, and can safely wait. Each facility should determine acceptable waiting times if a room is not immediately available. In assigning this acuity, the nurse should consider that the patient may need only a simple exam. To improve customer service, the nurse should reassess the waiting patient, per facility protocol, and offer comfort measures.

Nursing Considerations: In addition to assigning acuity based on symptoms and resources needed, the nurse is prompted when appropriate to initiate certain nursing interventions. Nurses should initiate only those nursing interventions that have been approved by their facilities.

Relevant Protocols: This section lists additional protocols to consider that may assist in determining a more appropriate patient disposition.

Appendices

This section provides additional information to support the protocols, broaden the nurse's scope of knowledge, and prompt the nurse to look further in identifying potentially lethal conditions.

Appendix A: The PQRSTT mnemonic assessment guide assists the nurse in asking the questions that will result in a comprehensive and high-quality interview.

Appendices B, C, D, E, F: Provide quick reference charts to determine the appropriate dosages for acetaminophen and ibuprofen, as well as weight and temperature conversions.

Appendices G, H, I: Provide additional information about three symptoms that are potentially life-threatening: abdominal pain, chest pain, and headaches. While nurses do not diagnose, it is important that they understand the conditions and symptoms that may be lethal.

Appendices J, K, L, M, N: Address mechanism of injury (MOI) by age group. This handy guide describes the types of injuries the nurse could anticipate based on age and MOI. This information will help to alert the nurse to potentially lethal conditions that initially could go undetected.

Appendix O: A comprehensive reference tool on the most commonly used, abused, and recreational drugs, their common names, and their effects.

Appendix P: A good reference on the signs and symptoms of the most common types of poisoning.

Appendix Q: A handy reference on the biological and chemical agents most commonly anticipated to be used in a terrorist attack. The triage nurse may be the first to recognize the symptoms or a pattern and should report findings to the appropriate authority, per facility policy.

Appendix R: A comprehensive chart describing the most common communicable diseases, cold vs. flu symptoms, and STDs. Includes modes of transmission, incubation periods, and contagious periods.

Appendix S: A triage assessment form to use as a model in evaluating nurses' interactions with patients.

Appendix T: A set of training exercises to aid nurses in identifying appropriate interventions at triage and identifying risk factors that might have an impact on assignment of acuity level.

Additional Triage Guidelines

While every effort was made to design each protocol in the most comprehensive manner possible to be age-specific and reflective of high-risk patients, the triage nurse should be aware of the many factors that impact the severity of symptoms, the appropriate triage disposition, and the triage experience:

- Ages >65 and <1 month
- Comorbidities, smoking, obesity, chronic disease, alcohol or drug use/abuse, immunosuppression, hypertension, sedentary life style
- Mechanism of injury (see appendices for age-specific guidelines)
- Continued assessment while waiting
- Potential EMTALA violations (all patients have a right to a medical screening— review the facility's EMTALA policies)

In addition, the triage nurse should:

- Develop and use standing orders to facilitate treatment/diagnostic interventions at triage to improve patient satisfaction and throughput.
- Keep patients informed while waiting—use this opportunity to continually reassess and improve customer satisfaction.
- Monitor consistency in applying triage criteria and assigning acuity.
- Train staff in use of protocols with the 5-tier triage system.
- Create scenarios to rate consistency in the application of triage protocols.

Julie K. Briggs, RN, BSN, MHA
Valerie G. A. Grossman, BSN, CEN

Acknowledgments

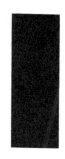

This has been a great experience and opportunity to work together from across the country in the creation of this worthwhile project. We would like to express our gratitude and appreciation to Marge Bentler, RN, BSN, CEN, Dr. Bret Lambert and Dr. Michael Brook for their thorough review and suggestions. We would also like to extend a special thank you to Theresa Tavernero, RN, BSN, CEN, MHA, for her interest, contributions and insightful suggestions for developing a quality product.

Julie Briggs and Valerie Grossman

Additionally, I would like to thank Valerie Grossman, my husband Worth, and my parents and friends for their continued support and encouragement throughout this project, as I struggled to balance deadlines and life's unforeseeable challenges.

Julie

I am honored to have worked on this book with Julie, who has been a friend and mentor for many years. My sincere appreciation goes to my daughters (Sarah and Nicole), my sister (Christina), and my parents (John and Marie), who support my every project . . . and to Senior Chief Petty Officer Scott D. Grossman, US Navy, for wherever he is in the world, he is always a role model for our family to emulate.

Valerie

Contents

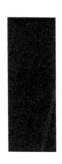

Bibliography, 177

Appendices

Abdominal Pain, Adult

? KEY QUESTIONS:

Name • Age • Onset • Allergies • Prior History • Associated Symptoms • Pain Scale • Description and Location of the Pain • Vital Signs • Medications

Acuity Level/Assessment	Nursing Considerations
●●● Level 1: Critical	**Resuscitation**
Pale, diaphoretic, and confused or weak Unresponsive Apnea or severe respiratory distress Pulseless	**Immediate treatment** Many resources needed Staff at bedside Mobilization of resuscitation team
●●● Level 2: High Risk	**Emergent**
Penetrating wound to abdomen New-onset, rapidly increasing pain in abdomen radiating to back or legs and age >50 yr Vomiting large amount of blood Lightheadedness Sudden-onset severe pain and abnormal vital signs Signs and symptoms of dehydration Age >50 yr and systolic BP <100 Bloody stools (unrelated to hemorrhoids or rectal fissure) Vaginal bleeding saturating more than three regular-size pads per hour History of fainting episodes Altered mental status	**Do not delay treatment** Notify physician Nothing by mouth until examined Do not remove protruding object if present Multiple diagnostic studies or procedures Frequent consultation Constant monitoring
●●● Level 3: Moderate Risk	**Urgent**
Severe pain Heavy vaginal bleeding and possibility of pregnancy Sudden onset Constipation and fever >101°F (38.3°C)	**Refer for treatment as soon as possible** Nothing by mouth until examined Monitor for change in condition May need multiple diagnostic studies or procedures

Acuity Level/Assessment	Nursing Considerations
Level 3: Moderate Risk	**Urgent**
Vomiting dark, coffee-ground–like emesis Vomiting and abdominal distention Pregnancy Rapidly increasing pain Right lower quadrant pain with poor appetite, nausea or vomiting, or fever Ingestion of plant, drug, or chemical Age >65 yr	If vital signs abnormal, consider Level 2
Level 4: Low Risk	**Semi-Urgent**
Black tarry stools with foul odor History of recent abdominal surgery or chronic pain Nausea and vomiting Fever >101°F (38.3°C) Continuous pain >1 hour Painful or difficult urination Blood in urine Unexplained progressive abdominal swelling	Reassess while waiting, per facility protocol Nothing by mouth until examined Offer comfort measures May need simple diagnostic study or procedure
Level 5: Lower Risk	Non-Urgent
No other symptoms, but parent/patient concerned Intermittent pain Overconsumption of foods or fluids Flatulence Sensation of bladder fullness	Reassess while waiting, per facility protocol Offer comfort measures May need examination only

RELATED PROTOCOLS:

Diarrhea, Adult • Foreign Body, Ingestion • Menstrual Problems • Poisoning, Exposure or Ingestion • Pregnancy, Abdominal Pain • Urination Problems • Vaginal Bleeding, Abnormal • Vomiting

See Appendix G: Differential Diagnosis of Abdominal Pain

Abdominal Pain, Child

Name • Age • Onset • Allergies • Prior History • Associated Symptoms • Pain Scale • Description and Location of the Pain • Vital Signs • Medications

Acuity Level/Assessment	Nursing Considerations
●●● **Level 1: Critical**	**Resuscitation**
Pale, diaphoretic, and confused, weak, or limp Apnea or severe respiratory distress Unresponsive Pulseless	**Immediate treatment** Many resources needed Staff at bedside Mobilization of resuscitation team
●●● **Level 2: High Risk**	**Emergent**
Altered mental status New-onset, rapidly increasing severe pain Grasping abdomen, walking bent over, screaming, or lying with knees drawn toward chest Ingestion of unknown chemical substance, plant, medication, or object Signs and symptoms of dehydration Penetrating wound to abdomen Severe pain >1 hr	**Do not delay treatment** Notify physician Do not remove protruding object if present Multiple diagnostic studies or procedures Frequent consultation Continuous monitoring Nothing by mouth until examined
●●● **Level 3: Moderate Risk**	**Urgent**
Possibility of pregnancy Sudden onset Fever >101°F (38.3°C) Age <2 yr and intermittent pain Recent abdominal trauma Right lower quadrant pain with poor appetite, nausea, vomiting, or fever Severe nausea or vomiting Bloody or jelly-like stools Black stools History of recent abdominal surgery	**Refer for treatment as soon as possible** May need multiple diagnostic studies or procedures Monitor for change in condition Nothing by mouth until examined If vital signs abnormal, consider Level 2

Acuity Level/Assessment	Nursing Considerations
Level 3: Moderate Risk	**Urgent**
Unable to comfort Suspected abuse	
Level 4: Low Risk	**Semi-Urgent**
Mild nausea and vomiting Painful or difficult urination Blood in urine	Reassess while waiting, per facility protocol Offer comfort measures Nothing by mouth until examined May need simple diagnostic study or procedure
Level 5: Lower Risk	Non-Urgent
Intermittent pain associated with eating, empty stomach, or use of pain, antibiotic, or anti-inflammatory medications Unexplained progressive abdominal swelling	Reassess while waiting, per facility protocol May need examination only Offer comfort measures

RELATED PROTOCOLS:

Constipation • Diarrhea • Foreign Body, Ingestion • Menstrual Problems • Poisoning, Exposure or Ingestion • Pregnancy, abdominal pain • Urination Problems • Vaginal Bleeding • Vomiting

See Appendix G: Differential Diagnosis of Abdominal Pain

Notes

Alcohol and Drug Use, Abuse, and Dependence

KEY QUESTIONS:

Name • Age • Onset • Allergies • Prior History • Medications • Pain Scale • Vital Signs • Drug or Drinking Habits • Amount and Frequency • Hours or Days Since Last Use or Drink

Acuity Level/Assessment	Nursing Considerations
Level 1: Critical	**Resuscitation**
Apnea or severe difficulty breathing Pale, diaphoretic, and lightheaded or weak Unresponsive Pulseless	**Immediate treatment** Many resources needed Staff at bedside Mobilization of resuscitation team
Level 2: High Risk	**Emergent**
Under the influence and rapid heart rate, chest pain, difficulty breathing, shakiness, dizziness Threat to hurt self or others Suicidal behavior Overdose Altered mental status	**Do not delay treatment** Notify physician Multiple diagnostic studies or procedures Frequent consultation Continuous monitoring Keep suicidal patient under observation
Level 3: Moderate Risk	**Urgent**
Palpitations Signs of withdrawal; rapid heartbeat, diaphoresis, fever, auditory or visual hallucinations or delusions Extremely anxious, sense of terror, agitation Severe pain New onset of hallucinations or paranoia Suicidal thoughts but no action	**Refer for treatment as soon as possible** Contact crisis worker, per facility policy Monitor for change in condition May need multiple diagnostic studies or procedures If abnormal vital signs, consider Level 2 Keep suicidal patient under observation

Acuity Level/Assessment	Nursing Considerations
Level 4: Low Risk	**Semi-Urgent**
Hyperventilation Profuse sweating Acute anxiety Distorted perceptions Difficulty functioning	Provide bag and hyperventilation instructions as necessary Reassess while waiting, per facility protocol Offer comfort measures May need a simple diagnostic study or procedure Maintain visual contact of patient
Level 5: Lower Risk	Non-Urgent
No physical symptoms History of intermittent use and parent wants patient tested Request for help with addiction	Reassess while waiting, per facility protocol Offer comfort measures May need an examination only May need social worker consult

RELATED PROTOCOLS:
Altered Mental Status • Anxiety • Chest Pain

See Appendix O: Drugs of Abuse

Notes

Allergic Reaction

KEY QUESTIONS:

Name • Age • Onset • Allergies • Prior History • Severity • Pain Scale • Suspected Cause • Vital Signs • Oxygen Saturation • Medications

Acuity Level/Assessment	Nursing Considerations
Level 1: Critical	**Resuscitation**
Severe difficulty breathing Unresponsive Pale, diaphoretic, lightheaded, or weak Unable to speak Severe swelling of tongue or throat Hypotension O_2 saturation <90% with oxygen	**Immediate treatment** Staff at bedside Mobilization of resuscitation team Many resources needed
Level 2: High Risk	**Emergent**
Moderate oral swelling Audible stridor or wheezing Hoarse voice Moderate respiratory distress Speaking in short words Prior anaphylaxis requiring epinephrine Difficulty swallowing Chest pain Rapid progression of symptoms Altered mental status Urticaria and hives throughout body O_2 saturation <94% with oxygen O_2 saturation <90% on room air	**Do not delay treatment** Notify physician Multiple diagnostic studies or procedures Frequent consultation Continuous monitoring
Level 3: Moderate Risk	**Urgent**

Symptoms persist after administration of
    Benadryl or epinephrine
Minimal oral swelling
Mild respiratory distress
Speaking in partial sentences
	Refer for treatment as soon as possible
	Monitor for change in condition
	May need a breathing treatment while waiting
	May need multiple diagnostic studies or
	    procedures

Acuity Level/Assessment	Nursing Considerations
Level 3: Moderate Risk	**Urgent**
Persistent nausea, vomiting, or diarrhea Urticaria >50% of body Fever or severe pain	If vital signs abnormal, consider Level 2
Level 4: Low Risk	**Semi-Urgent**
Dermal contact with allergen Speaking in full sentences Urticaria in large, localized area Moderate pain	Reassess while waiting, per facility protocol Offer comfort measures May need a simple diagnostic study or procedure
Level 5: Lower Risk	Non-Urgent
Persistent rash No respiratory problems Suspect medication reaction Urticaria in small localized area Minimal swelling in face or extremities	Reassess while waiting, per facility protocol Offer comfort measures May need an examination only

RELATED PROTOCOLS:

Asthma • Bee Sting • Breathing Problems • Hives

Notes

Altered Mental Status

Name • Age • Onset • Allergies • Medications • Prior History • Severity • Pain Scale • Vital Signs • Oxygen Saturation

Acuity Level/Assessment	Nursing Considerations
Level 1: Critical	**Resuscitation**
Apnea or severe respiratory distress Unresponsive Pale, diaphoretic, and lightheaded or weak Status epilepticus Pulseless	**Refer for immediate treatment** Staff at bedside Mobilization of resuscitation team Many resources needed
Level 2: High Risk	**Emergent**
Altered mental status Drug or alcohol overdose Danger to self or others Severe headache Chest pain Rapid heartbeat with syncope/diaphoresis Abnormal vital signs (HR<50 or >100, R<8) Diabetic Pregnancy and heavy vaginal bleeding or abdominal pain Severe abdominal pain Loss of movement in arms or legs, confusion, difficulty speaking, numbness, tingling or blurred vision, and onset <2 hr ago Extreme agitation or restlessness Headache and projectile vomiting Headache, fever, and stiff or painful neck Hallucinations, delusions, or mania	**Do not delay treatment** Notify physician Multiple diagnostic studies or procedures Frequent consultation Continuous monitoring

Acuity Level/Assessment	Nursing Considerations
Level 3: Moderate Risk	**Urgent**
Person is arousable, oriented, and any of the following: Headache, fever without stiff or painful neck Recent head injury or trauma (rule out head bleed) New seizure and prolonged postictal state Persistent high fever Severe abdominal pain and normal vital signs Temporary slurred speech or weakened grips Tonic or clonic seizure Recently ingested pain, cold, or sleeping medication	**Refer for treatment as soon as possible** May need multiple diagnostic studies or procedures Monitor for change in condition If vital signs abnormal, consider Level 2
Level 4: Low Risk	**Semi-Urgent**
Brief period of loss of consciousness Alcohol intoxication Recreational drug use	Offer comfort measures Reassess while waiting, per facility protocol May need simple diagnostic study or procedure
Level 5: Lower Risk	Non-Urgent
Exhaustion Sleep deprivation	Offer comfort measures Reassess while waiting, per facility protocol May need examination only

RELATED PROTOCOLS:
Alcohol and Drug Use, Abuse, and Dependence • Breathing Problems • Chest Pain • Fever • Headache
• Head Injury

Ankle Pain and Swelling (nontraumatic; for injury, see Extremity Injury)

Acuity Level/Assessment	Nursing Considerations
●●● **Level 1: Critical**	**Resuscitation**
Ankle swelling and severe difficulty breathing	**Immediate treatment** Staff at bedside Mobilization of resuscitation team Many resources needed
●●● **Level 2: High Risk**	**Emergent**
Chest pain Coughing blood New onset and unable to walk No pedal pulse in affected extremity Foot pale, cold, or blue compared to other foot Severe pain Altered mental status	**Do not delay treatment** Notify physician Multiple diagnostic studies or procedures Frequent consultation Continuous monitoring
●●● **Level 3: Moderate Risk**	**Urgent**
Swelling and pain in ankle, thigh, or calf Pain or swelling and fever Area over ankle, calf, or thigh hot/warm to touch or red Sudden swelling and tenderness in single leg or ankle Foot numb compared to other foot Difficulty walking Pregnancy and sudden weight gain	**Refer for treatment as soon as possible** Monitor for change in condition May need multiple diagnostic studies or procedures If vital signs abnormal, consider Level 2

Acuity Level/Assessment	Nursing Considerations
Level 4: Low Risk	**Semi-Urgent**
Pain in the joint or base of the big toe Red and shiny skin over the joint	Reassess while waiting, per facility protocol Offer comfort measures May need a simple diagnostic study or 　procedure
Level 5: Lower Risk	Non-Urgent
Pregnancy and gradual weight gain	Reassess while waiting, per facility protocol Offer comfort measures May need an examination only

RELATED PROTOCOLS:
Extremity Injury

Notes

Anxiety
(if chest pain is present, see Chest Pain)

Acuity Level/Assessment	Nursing Considerations
●●● **Level 1: Critical**	**Resuscitation**
Severe difficulty breathing Pale, diaphoretic and lightheaded or weak	**Immediate treatment** Many resources needed Staff at bedside Mobilization of resuscitation team
●●● **Level 2: High Risk**	**Emergent**
New onset of hallucinations or paranoia Confusion Suicidal behavior Overdose Altered mental status	**Do not delay treatment** Notify physician Multiple diagnostic studies or procedures Frequent consultation Continuous monitoring
●●● **Level 3: Moderate Risk**	**Urgent**
Palpitations Difficulty functioning Extremely anxious Severe pain	**Refer for treatment as soon as possible** Contact crisis worker, per facility policy Monitor for change in condition May need multiple diagnostic studies or procedures If abnormal vital signs, consider Level 2
●●● **Level 4: Low Risk**	**Semi-Urgent**
Hyperventilation Profuse sweating Persistent upset stomach Emotional or situational stress Increased caffeine consumption	Provide bag and hyperventilation instructions as necessary Reassess while waiting, per facility protocol Offer comfort measures May need a simple diagnostic study or procedure

Acuity Level/Assessment	Nursing Considerations
Level 5: Lower Risk	Non-Urgent
No physical symptoms History of anxiety episodes and now asymptomatic	Reassess while waiting, per facility protocol Offer comfort measures May need an examination only

RELATED PROTOCOLS:

Breathing Problems • Chest Pain

Notes

Asthma

KEY QUESTIONS:

Name • Age • Onset • Allergies • Prior Asthma History • Severity • Duration • Prior Treatment • Medications • Pain Scale • Vital Signs • Oxygen Saturation • Peak Flow Meter Measurement

Acuity Level/Assessment	Nursing Considerations
●●● **Level 1: Critical**	**Resuscitation**
Apnea or severe respiratory distress Unable to speak Central cyanosis Unresponsive Pale, diaphoretic, lightheaded, or weak O_2 saturation <90% with oxygen	**Immediate treatment** Staff at bedside Mobilization of resuscitation team Many resources needed
●●● **Level 2: High Risk**	**Emergent**
Speaking in short words Use of accessory muscles and fatigue Sudden onset of wheezing after medication, food, bee sting, or exposure to known allergen Peak flow rate <50% of baseline Altered mental status Chest pain O_2 saturation <94% with oxygen O_2 saturation <90% on room air Heightened anxiety, fear, or restlessness	**Do not delay treatment** Notify physician Multiple diagnostic studies or procedures Frequent consultation Continuous monitoring
●●● **Level 3: Moderate Risk**	**Urgent**
Speaking in partial sentences Severe cough Prior hospitalization for same symptoms Persistent, audible wheezing 20 min after treatment Fever >103°F (39.4°C)	**Refer for treatment as soon as possible** Monitor for change in condition May need a breathing treatment while waiting May need multiple diagnostic studies or procedures If abnormal vital signs, consider Level 2

Acuity Level/Assessment	Nursing Considerations
Level 4: Low Risk	**Semi-Urgent**
Speaking in full sentences Persistent cough after use of inhaler or nebulizer Fever <103°F (39.4°C) Age >60 yr and fever >101°F (38.3°C) Peak flow rate >80% of baseline	Reassess while waiting, per facility protocol Offer comfort measures May need a simple diagnostic study or procedure
Level 5: Lower Risk	Non-Urgent
Fever and green or yellow nasal discharge Resolution of wheezing after use of inhaler or nebulizer Peak flow back to baseline	Reassess while waiting, per facility protocol Offer comfort measures May need an examination only

RELATED PROTOCOLS:
Allergic Reaction • Breathing Problems • Cough

Notes

Back Pain

KEY QUESTIONS:

Name • Age • Onset • Allergies • Prior History • Severity • Pain Scale • Vital Signs • Medications

Acuity Level/Assessment	Nursing Considerations
● ● ● Level 1: Critical	**Resuscitation**
Apnea or severe respiratory distress Unresponsive Pulseless Pale, diaphoretic, and lightheaded or weak Recent trauma and unable to move toes or severe weakness in one or both lower extremities	**Refer for immediate treatment** Staff at bedside Mobilization of resuscitation team Many resources needed
● ● ● Level 2: High Risk	**Emergent**
Altered mental status New-onset, rapidly increasing pain and age >60 yr New-onset loss of sensation to lower extremities Progressive weakness in legs Loss of bladder or bowel control Penetrating trauma to back or flank	**Refer for treatment within minutes** Notify physician Multiple diagnostic studies or procedures Frequent consultation Continuous monitoring Do not remove penetrating object
● ● ● Level 3: Moderate Risk	**Urgent**
Severe back or abdominal pain New-onset numbness and tingling in legs Hematuria and severe abdominal or flank pain Hematuria and blunt trauma to the back or flank Pain with urination and fever >100.5°F (38.1°C) or chills New-onset, rapidly increasing pain and age <60 yr	**Refer for treatment as soon as possible** Monitor for change in condition May need multiple diagnostic studies or procedures If abnormal vital signs, consider Level 2

Acuity Level/Assessment	Nursing Considerations
●●● **Level 3: Moderate Risk**	**Urgent**
History of diabetes, immunosuppression, or intravenous drug abuse Unable to urinate >8 hr Male with fever and nausea or vomiting History of disk injury or back surgery	
●●● **Level 4: Low Risk**	**Semi-Urgent**
Trauma within past week and worsening pain, numbness, tingling, or weakness in extremity Pain restricting ability to walk Age <65 yr Pain increasing with activity Pain radiating to buttocks or hips	Reassess while waiting, per facility protocol Offer comfort measures May need simple diagnostic study or procedure
●●● Level 5: Lower Risk	Non-Urgent
Chronic low back pain Minor discomfort Rash over the painful area	Reassess while waiting, per facility protocol Offer comfort measures May need an examination only

RELATED PROTOCOLS:

Motor Vehicle Accident • Neck Pain • Urination Problems

Bee Sting

Name • Age • Onset • Allergies • Prior History • Severity • Pain Scale • Vital Signs • Oxygen Saturation • Previous Bee Sting Reaction and Treatment

Acuity Level/Assessment	Nursing Considerations
Level 1: Critical	**Resuscitation**
Apnea or severe difficulty breathing Unresponsive Pale, diaphoretic, and lightheaded or weak Hypotension Unable to speak Severe swelling of tongue or throat O_2 saturation <90% with oxygen	**Immediate treatment** Staff at bedside Mobilization of resuscitation team Many resources needed
Level 2: High Risk	**Emergent**
Moderate oral swelling Audible stridor or wheezing Hoarse voice Moderate respiratory distress Speaking in short words Prior anaphylaxis requiring epinephrine Difficulty swallowing Chest pain Rapid progression of symptoms Altered mental status Urticaria and hives throughout body Bee sting in the mouth O_2 saturation <94% with oxygen O_2 saturation <90% on room air	**Do not delay treatment** Notify physician Multiple diagnostic studies or procedures Frequent consultation Continuous monitoring
Level 3: Moderate Risk	**Urgent**
Speaking in partial sentences Nausea, vomiting, or weakness >10 stings Generalized hives after Benadryl or epinephrine	**Refer for treatment as soon as possible** Monitor for changes in condition May need multiple diagnostic studies or procedures

Acuity Level/Assessment	Nursing Considerations
●●● **Level 3: Moderate Risk**	**Urgent**

Mild wheezing
Minimal reaction to bee sting and:
    Prior anaphylaxis requiring epinephrine
    Bee sting in the mouth
	If abnormal vital signs, consider Level 2

●●● **Level 4: Low Risk**	**Semi-Urgent**

Able to speak in full sentences
Urticaria or rash locations other than sting site
Signs of infection: drainage, fever, red streaks,
    or pus 24–48 hrs after the sting
	Reassess while waiting, per facility protocol
	Offer comfort measures
	May need a simple diagnostic study or
	    procedure

●●● Level 5: Lower Risk	Non-Urgent
Localized swelling, pain, or urticaria around sting site	Reassess while waiting, per facility protocol Offer comfort measures May need an examination only

RELATED PROTOCOLS:

Allergic Reaction • Bites, Insect and Tick • Breathing Problems • Hives

Notes

Bites, Animal and Human

Name • Age • Onset • Location • Allergies • Prior History • Severity • Pain Scale • Vital Signs • Tetanus Immunization Status

Acuity Level/Assessment	Nursing Considerations
●●● **Level 1: Critical**	**Resuscitation**
Apnea or severe respiratory distress Pulseless Unresponsive	**Refer for immediate treatment** Many resources needed Staff at bedside Mobilization of resuscitation team
●●● **Level 2: High Risk**	**Emergent**
Altered mental status Pulsatile bleeding Multiple gaping wounds Difficulty breathing or swallowing	**Do not delay treatment** Notify physician Multiple diagnostic studies or procedures Frequent consultation Constant monitoring
●●● **Level 3: Moderate Risk**	**Urgent**
Severe pain Gaping wounds	**Refer for treatment as soon as possible** May need multiple diagnostic studies or procedures Monitor for changes in condition If vital signs abnormal, consider Level 2
●●● **Level 4: Low Risk**	**Semi-Urgent**

Moderate pain
Stable wounds
Abrasive wounds
Signs of infection: drainage, fever, red streaks,
    or pus >24 hr after the bite
History of chronic illness
Controlled bleeding
Risk for rabies exposure
	Reassess while waiting, per facility protocol
	Offer comfort measures
	May need a simple diagnostic study or
	    procedure

Acuity Level/Assessment	Nursing Considerations
Level 5: Lower Risk	Non-Urgent
No break in skin Tetanus status unknown or booster >5 yr	Reassess while waiting, per facility protocol Offer comfort measures May need examination only

RELATED PROTOCOLS:
Laceration • Puncture Wound • Wound Infection

Notes

_____
_____
_____
_____
_____
_____
_____
_____
_____
_____
_____
_____
_____
_____
_____
_____
_____
_____
_____

Bites, Insect and Tick

Acuity Level/Assessment	Nursing Considerations
Level 1: Critical	**Resuscitation**
Apnea or severe respiratory distress Pulseless Unresponsive Hypotension Unable to speak Severe swelling of tongue or throat Unable to swallow, drooling	**Refer for immediate treatment** Many resources needed Staff at bedside Mobilization of resuscitation team
Level 2: High Risk	**Emergent**
Altered mental status Speaking in short words Difficulty breathing or chest pain Swelling of tongue or mouth with difficulty swallowing Urticaria and hives throughout body	**Do not delay treatment** Notify physician Multiple diagnostic studies or procedures Frequent consultation Constant monitoring
Level 3: Moderate Risk	**Urgent**
Severe pain Speaking in partial sentences Prior anaphylaxis to insect bite requiring epinephrine Widespread hives Numerous bites, stings, or ticks Flu-like symptoms with a history of tick bite 2 to 4 wk previous Brown recluse spider bite Black widow spider and no other symptoms	**Refer for treatment as soon as possible** May need multiple diagnostic studies or procedures Monitor for changes in condition If vital signs abnormal, consider Level 2

Acuity Level/Assessment	Nursing Considerations
Level 4: Low Risk	**Semi-Urgent**
Moderate pain Signs of infection: fever, red streaks, pus, or drainage >24 hr after bite Unable to remove tick or tick head remains under skin Peeling skin around the site	Reassess while waiting, per facility protocol Offer comfort measures May need a simple diagnostic study or procedure
Level 5: Lower Risk	Non-Urgent
Sporadic hives	Reassess while waiting, per facility protocol Offer comfort measures May need examination only

RELATED PROTOCOLS:
Allergic Reaction • Laceration • Wound Infection

Notes

Bites, Marine Animal

Name • Age • Onset • Allergies • Prior History • Severity • Pain Scale • Vital Signs • Tetanus Immunization Status • Marine Animal Identification

Acuity Level/Assessment	Nursing Considerations
●●● **Level 1: Critical**	**Resuscitation**
Apnea or severe difficulty breathing Unresponsive Pale, diaphoretic, and lightheaded or weak Hypotension Unable to speak	**Immediate treatment** Staff at bedside Mobilization of resuscitation team Many resources needed
●●● **Level 2: High Risk**	**Emergent**
Altered mental status Pulsatile bleeding Limb amputation Chest pain or difficulty breathing Swelling of throat, tongue, lips Loss of pulses distal to injury	**Do not delay treatment** Notify physician Multiple diagnostic studies or procedures Frequent consultation Continuous monitoring
●●● **Level 3: Moderate Risk**	**Urgent**
Severe pain Diaphoretic Pallor Hives Extremity swelling Vision changes Prior anaphylaxis requiring epinephrine	**Refer for treatment as soon as possible** Monitor for changes in condition May need multiple diagnostic studies or procedures If abnormal vital signs, consider Level 2
●●● **Level 4: Low Risk**	**Semi-Urgent**
Moderate pain Stung by Portuguese man-of-war jellyfish Decreased range of motion Stinger present	Reassess while waiting, per facility protocol Offer comfort measures For catfish, lionfish, scorpion fish, sea urchin, stingrays, starfish, stone fish, and

Acuity Level/Assessment	Nursing Considerations
●●● **Level 4: Low Risk**	**Semi-Urgent**
	surgeonfish spine punctures: consider soaking injured part in hot saltwater for 30 to 90 min for pain relief while waiting May need a simple diagnostic study or procedure
●●● Level 5: Lower Risk	Non-Urgent
History of non-poisonous bite with no signs or symptoms Tetanus status unknown or booster >5 yr	Reassess while waiting, per facility protocol Offer comfort measures May need an examination only

RELATED PROTOCOLS:

Allergic Reaction • Laceration • Puncture Wound • Wound Infection

Notes

Bites, Snake

KEY QUESTIONS:
Name • Age • Onset • Location • Allergies • Prior History • Severity • Pain Scale • Vital Signs • Tetanus Immunization Status • Type of Snake

Acuity Level/Assessment	Nursing Considerations
●●● **Level 1: Critical**	**Resuscitation**
Apnea or severe difficulty breathing Unresponsive Pale, diaphoretic, and lightheaded or weak Hypotension Unable to speak Severe swelling of tongue or throat O_2 saturation <90% with oxygen	**Refer for immediate treatment** Many resources needed Staff at bedside Mobilization of resuscitation team
●●● **Level 2: High Risk**	**Emergent**
Altered mental status Bite from a poisonous snake, such as rattlesnake, copperhead, water moccasin, or coral snake Chest pain Difficulty swallowing or breathing	**Do not delay treatment** Notify physician Multiple diagnostic studies or procedures Frequent consultation Constant monitoring
●●● **Level 3: Moderate Risk**	**Urgent**

Severe pain
Puncture wound(s) from unidentified snake
Purple rash, fever, pallor, or facial numbness or
    tingling
Prior anaphylaxis to snake bite requiring
    epinephrine
	Refer for treatment as soon as possible
	May need multiple diagnostic studies or
	    procedures
	Monitor for change in condition
	If vital signs abnormal, consider Level 2

●●● **Level 4: Low Risk**	**Semi-Urgent**

Moderate pain
Multiple bites from nonpoisonous snake
Signs of local infection: drainage, fever, red
    streaks, or pus >24 hr after bite
Swelling around the wound
	Reassess while waiting, per facility protocol
	Offer comfort measures
	May need a simple diagnostic study or
	    procedure

Acuity Level/Assessment	Nursing Considerations
Level 5: Lower Risk	Non-Urgent
Need for updated tetanus immunization	Reassess while waiting, per facility protocol Offer comfort measures May need examination only

RELATED PROTOCOLS:
Allergic Reaction • Laceration • Wound Infection

Notes

Body Art Complications

KEY QUESTIONS:

Name • Age • Onset • Allergies • Prior History (Including Infectious Diseases) • Severity • Pain Scale • Vital Signs • Oximetry • Location of Body Art • Performed by Whom (Professional Versus Amateur) • When Performed • Immunizations (dT, Hep B)

Acuity Level/Assessment	Nursing Considerations
●●● **Level 1: Critical**	**Resuscitation**
Apnea or severe respiratory distress Pulseless Unresponsive Pale, diaphoretic, and lightheaded or weak	**Refer for immediate treatment** Staff at bedside Mobilization of resuscitation team Many resources needed Remove piercings that interfere with c-spine stabilization, medical antishock trousers, intubation, Sager splint, Foley catheter, or defibrillator Avoid using wire cutters to remove piercings
●●● **Level 2: High Risk**	**Emergent**
Altered mental status Fever, hypotension, tachycardia, weakness Chest pain Piercing torn from site and unable to stop bleeding with pressure	**Do not delay treatment** Notify physician Multiple diagnostic studies or procedures Frequent consultation Continuous monitoring Remove piercings that interfere with c-spine stabilization, medical antishock trousers, intubation, Sager splint, foley catheter or defibrillation Avoid using wire cutters to remove piercings
●●● **Level 3: Moderate Risk**	**Urgent**
Severe pain Skin reddened, peeling off in sheets Skin red and warm to touch and fever Fever, chills, general malaise, or headache Vomiting, abdominal pain, jaundice	**Refer for treatment as soon as possible** May need multiple diagnostic studies or procedures Monitor for change in condition Leave piercing in place if possible

Acuity Level/Assessment	Nursing Considerations
●●● **Level 3: Moderate Risk**	**Urgent**
Piercing torn from site, bleeding controlled Swallowed oral jewelry Swollen lymph nodes and fever	If vital signs abnormal, consider Level 2
●●● **Level 4: Low Risk**	**Semi-Urgent**

Moderate pain
Skin red and warm to touch, swelling, or red
    streaks (no fever)
Jewelry slipped inside of piercing site, no
    visible jewelry
Swollen lymph node
Darkened hard and painful area around the
    piercing or tattoo
	Reassess while waiting, per facility protocol
	Offer comfort measures
	May need simple diagnostic study or procedure
	Leave piercing in place if possible

●●● Level 5: Lower Risk	Non-Urgent

Body art remorse (patient or parent requests
    reversal of procedure)
No other symptoms, but new piercing or
    tattoo and patient or parent concerned
	Reassess while waiting, per facility protocol
	Offer comfort measures
	May need examination only

RELATED PROTOCOLS:
Laceration • Wound Infection

Common Complications: Body Piercing

Location	Jewelry Used	Healing Time	Common Complications
Ampallang	Barbell stud	6 to 12 mo	• Keloid formation • May interrupt the flow of urine (may need to sit to void) • Formation of abscesses, cysts, or boils • Ripping and tearing of skin if jewelry gets caught on clothing
Cheek	Labret stud	6 to 8 wk	• Swelling, infection, gum injury, increased salivation • Chipped or broken teeth • Speech impairment

Common Complications: Body Piercing (continued)

Location	Jewelry Used	Healing Time	Common Complications
Cheek (continued)	Labret stud	6 to 8 wk	• Aspiration or ingestion of loosened jewelry • Difficulty chewing and swallowing • Massive systemic infection, septic shock • Formation of abscesses, cysts, or boils
Clitoris	Captive bead ring, barbell stud	4 to 10 wk	• Keloid formation • Formation of abscesses, cysts, or boils • Ripping and tearing of skin if jewelry gets caught on clothing
Clitoris hood	Captive bead ring, captive stone ring, circular barbell	4 to 10 wk	• Keloid formation • Formation of abscesses, cysts, or boils • Ripping and tearing of skin if jewelry gets caught on clothing
Earlobe	Captive bead ring, circular barbell, captive stone ring	4 to 6 wk	• Keloid formation • Formation of abscesses, cysts, or boils • Ripping and tearing of skin if jewelry gets caught on clothing
Ear cartilage	Same pieces as an earlobe; larger gauge is used	4 to 12 mo	• Keloid formation • Formation of abscesses, cysts, or boils • Prone to pseudomonal infections • Ripping and tearing of skin if jewelry gets caught on clothing
Ear plug	Increasing sizes of an object	Gradual enlargement of lobe	• Keloid formation • Overstretching of skin
Eyebrow	Captive bead ring, captive stone ring, barbell studs	6 to 8 wk	• Keloid formation • Ripping and tearing of skin if jewelry gets caught on clothing • Formation of abscesses, cysts, or boils • Excess hair growth over piercing area • Development of cysts • Periorbital cellulitis

Common Complications: Body Piercing (continued)

Location	Jewelry Used	Healing Time	Common Complications
Foreskin	Captive bead ring, captive stone ring, circular barbell	6 to 8 wk	• Formation of abscesses, cysts, or boils • Ripping and tearing of skin if jewelry gets caught on clothing • Keloid formation
Frenum	Barbell stud	6 to 8 wk	• Formation of abscesses, cysts, or boils • Ripping and tearing of skin if jewelry gets caught on clothing
Hand web	Captive bead ring, captive stone ring, barbell studs	6 to 12 mo	• Difficult healing, due to high rate of infection • Formation of abscesses, cysts, or boils • Ripping and tearing of skin if jewelry gets caught on clothing
Implants	Captive bead ring, captive stone ring, barbell studs, circular barbell, assorted other items (beads, spikes, coral, etc.)	2 to 4 mo	• Pressure on nerves, blood vessels, and muscles • Radiating pain that continues after healing complete • Shifting (when the object moves from its intended place) • Rejection by the body's immune system • Excess hair growth over implantation area • Formation of abscesses, cysts, or boils
Labia majora	Captive bead ring, captive stone ring, circular barbell	6 to 10 wk	• Keloid formation • Formation of abscesses, cysts, or boils • Ripping and tearing of skin if jewelry gets caught on clothing
Labia minora	Captive bead ring, captive stone ring, circular barbell	6 to 10 wk	• Keloid formation • Formation of abscesses, cysts, or boils • Ripping and tearing of skin if jewelry gets caught on clothing
Lip	Captive bead ring, captive stone ring, barbell studs	2 to 3 mo	• Swelling, infection, gingival injury, increased salivation • Keloid formation • Excess hair growth over pierced area

Common Complications: Body Piercing (continued)

Location	Jewelry Used	Healing Time	Common Complications
Lip (continued)	Captive bead ring, captive stone ring, barbell studs	2 to 3 mo	• Chipped or broken teeth • Speech impairment • Aspiration or ingestion of loosened jewelry • Massive systemic infection, septic shock • Formation of abscesses, cysts, or boils • Ripping and tearing of skin if jewelry gets caught on clothing
Nasal septum	Captive bead ring, circular barbell, septum retainer	2 to 8 mo	• Formation of abscesses, cysts, or boils • Ripping and tearing of skin if jewelry gets caught on clothing

Navel	Captive bead ring, captive stone ring, circular barbell	4 to 12 mo	• Very slow to heal: redness of area can last for months
			• Keloid formation
			• Excess hair growth over pierced area
			• Very high rate of infection (compared to other piercings) because of:
			  • constant friction, rubbing, and movement, and
			  • a bacteria-friendly environment (warm, dark, and moist)
			• Formation of abscesses, cysts, or boils
			• Ripping and tearing of skin if jewelry gets caught on clothing

Nipples (female)	Captive bead ring, captive stone ring, circular barbell	3 to 6 mo	• May damage some of the milk-producing ducts, causing mastitis or problems with future breast-feeding • Formation of abscesses, cysts, or boils • Ripping and tearing of skin if jewelry gets caught on clothing
Nipples (male)	Captive bead ring, captive stone ring, circular barbell	3 to 6 mo	• Formation of abscesses, cysts, or boils • Ripping and tearing of skin if jewelry gets caught on clothing

Common Complications: Body Piercing (continued)

Location	Jewelry Used	Healing Time	Common Complications
Nostril	Captive bead ring, captive stone ring	2 to 4 mo	• Keloid formation • Formation of abscesses, cysts, or boils • Ripping and tearing of skin if jewelry gets caught on clothing
Scrotum	Captive bead ring, captive stone ring, circular barbell	6 to 8 wk	• Ripping and tearing of skin if jewelry gets caught on clothing
Tongue	Barbell stud	4 to 6 wk	• Swelling, infection, gingival injury, increased salivation • Keloid formation • Chipped or broken teeth • Speech impairment • Aspiration or ingestion of loosened jewelry • Difficulty breathing, chewing, and swallowing • Prolonged bleeding • Massive systemic infection, septic shock • Damage to veins and nerves, including neuroma development
Tragus	Captive bead ring, circular barbell, captive stone ring	6 to 12 mo	• Formation of abscesses, cysts, or boils
Uvula	Captive bead ring, circular barbell, barbell stud	6 to 8 wk	• Swelling, infection, injury, increased salivation • Speech impairment • Aspiration or ingestion of loosened jewelry • Difficulty breathing and swallowing • Formation of abscesses, cysts, or boils

Breast Problems

KEY QUESTIONS:

Name • Age • Onset • Allergies • Prior History • Severity • Pain Scale • Vital Signs

Acuity Level/Assessment	Nursing Considerations
●●● **Level 1: Critical**	**Resuscitation**
Apnea or severe respiratory distress Unresponsive Pale, diaphoretic, and lightheaded or weak Hypotension	**Refer for immediate treatment** Many resources needed Staff at bedside Mobilization of resuscitation team
●●● **Level 2: High Risk**	**Emergent**
Altered mental status Difficulty breathing or chest pain	**Do not delay treatment** Notify physician Multiple diagnostic studies or procedures Frequent consultation Constant monitoring
●●● **Level 3: Moderate Risk**	**Urgent**
Severe pain Gaping lacerations	**Refer for treatment as soon as possible** May need multiple diagnostic studies or procedures Monitor for changes in condition If vital signs abnormal, consider Level 2
●●● **Level 4: Low Risk**	**Semi-Urgent**

Moderate pain
Skin ulceration
Bloody discharge
Foul-smelling discharge from nipples
Red, swollen, hot breasts
Trauma to breast
Signs of infection: drainage, fever, red streaks,
    or pus
	Reassess while waiting, per facility protocol
	Offer comfort measures
	May need a simple diagnostic study or
	    procedure

Acuity Level/Assessment	Nursing Considerations
Level 5: Lower Risk	Non-Urgent
Nipple discharge in non-pregnant woman Lump in breast unrelated to menstrual cycle Dimpling of breast tissue Lump in a male breast Unable to remove piercing	Reassess while waiting, per facility protocol Offer comfort measures May need examination only

RELATED PROTOCOLS:

Body Art Complications • Lacerations • Wound Infection

Notes

Breathing Problems

KEY QUESTIONS:
Name • Age • Weight • Onset • Allergies • Prior History • Severity • Pain Scale • Vital Signs • Oxygen Saturation • Medications

Acuity Level/Assessment	Nursing Considerations
●●● **Level 1: Critical**	**Resuscitation**
Apnea or severe respiratory distress Unresponsive Pulseless Unable to speak Central cyanosis O_2 saturation <90% with oxygen Severe retractions or acute cyanosis (Pediatric)	**Immediate treatment** Staff at bedside Mobilization of resuscitation team Many resources needed
●●● **Level 2: High Risk**	**Emergent**
Altered mental status Feeling of suffocation History of pulmonary embolus, blood clots, or lung collapse Chest pain Speaking in short words Pale skin or cyanotic fingernails Moderate retractions (Pediatric) Drooling O_2 saturation <94% with oxygen O_2 saturation <90% on room air Audible wheezes or severe stridor Diaphoresis Moderate use of accessory muscles Difficulty breathing and exposure to allergen that caused a significant reaction in the past Trauma and chest deformity	**Do not delay treatment** Notify physician Multiple diagnostic studies or procedures Frequent consultation Continuous monitoring Accurate O_2 saturation dependent upon good circulation and warm extremities Carbon monoxide poisoning will show adequate O_2 saturation in spite of poor oxygenation

Acuity Level/Assessment	Nursing Considerations
●●● **Level 3: Moderate Risk**	**Urgent**

Pain increasing with movement or breathing
Speaking in partial sentences
Mild, audible wheezes at rest
Tight cough
Frothy pink or copious white sputum
History of asthma not relieved with inhaler
Sudden or progressive shortness of breath and:
    Wheezing within past 2 hr;
    Recent trauma, surgery, or childbirth;
    Inhalation of a foreign body;
    Pallor; or
    High anxiety
	Refer for treatment as soon as possible
	Monitor for changes in condition
	May need a breathing treatment while waiting
	May need multiple diagnostic studies or
	    procedures
	If abnormal vital signs, consider Level 2

●●● **Level 4: Low Risk**	**Semi-Urgent**

Speaking in full sentences
Fever >103°F (39.4°C)
Productive cough with gray, green, or yellow
    sputum
Age >60 yr and fever >101°F (38.3°C)
	Reassess while waiting, per facility protocol
	Offer comfort measures
	May need a simple diagnostic study or
	    procedure

●●● Level 5: Lower Risk	Non-Urgent
O$_2$ saturation >95% on room air Occasional nonproductive cough Hyperventilation and numbness or tingling in fingers or face New stressful event or situation Exposure to environment irritant Recent cold or flu symptoms	Reassess while waiting, per facility protocol Offer comfort measures May need an examination only

RELATED PROTOCOLS:
Allergic Reaction • Asthma • Chest Pain • Foreign Body, Inhaled

Burns

KEY QUESTIONS:
Name • Age • Onset • Allergies • Medications • Prior History • Mechanism of Injury • Severity • Pain Scale • Vital Signs • Last Tetanus Immunization • Size and Location of Burn

Acuity Level/Assessment	Nursing Considerations
● ● ● Level 1: Critical	**Resuscitation**
Apnea or severe respiratory distress Pulseless Unresponsive Pale, diaphoretic, and lightheaded or weak	**Refer for immediate treatment** Staff at bedside Mobilization of resuscitation team Many resources needed
● ● ● Level 2: High Risk	**Emergent**
Altered mental status Extensive white and painless burn Extensive red and blistered burn and severe pain Difficulty breathing Chest pain or rapid irregular heartbeat Electrical or radiation burn Smoke inhalation with singed facial hair Burn circles neck extremity (and distal pulse)	**Do not delay treatment** Notify physician Multiple diagnostic studies or procedures Frequent consultation Continuous monitoring
● ● ● Level 3: Moderate Risk	**Urgent**
Severe pain Burned area charred (small area) Blistered or white painless burn > size of a hand Burn over a joint Blisters on face or neck Burn >1 inch and on face, eyes, ears, neck, hands, feet, or genital area	**Refer for treatment as soon as possible** Reassess, per facility protocol May need multiple diagnostic studies or procedures Monitor for changes in condition If vital signs abnormal, consider Level 2

Acuity Level/Assessment	Nursing Considerations
Level 4: Low Risk	**Semi-Urgent**
History of chronic illness Moderate pain Signs of infection Tetanus immunization >10 yr previous	Reassess while waiting, per facility protocol Offer comfort measures May need simple diagnostic study or procedure
Level 5: Lower Risk	Non-Urgent
Minimal pain Multiple open blisters	Reassess while waiting, per facility protocol Offer comfort measures May need examination only

RELATED PROTOCOLS:
Breathing Problems • Laceration • Poisoning, Exposure or Ingestion • Wound Infection

Notes

Chest Pain

Acuity Level/Assessment	Nursing Considerations
●●● Level 1: Critical	**Resuscitation**
Apnea or severe respiratory distress Unresponsive Pulseless Central cyanosis Hypotension	**Refer for immediate treatment** Staff at bedside Mobilization of resuscitation team Many resources needed
●●● Level 2: High Risk	**Emergent**
Altered mental status Lightheadedness or weakness Cool, moist skin Nausea or vomiting Pain radiates to neck, shoulders, jaw, back, or arms Age >35 yr and heart palpitations Difficulty breathing Skin pale Bilateral rales or rhonchi Persistent pain after 3 doses of nitroglycerin 5 min apart Known cardiac disease Severe chest pain at rest or awakens person Coughing up blood History of recent trauma, childbirth, or surgery Recreational street drug or prescription drug abuse within past 24 hr History of heart disease, diabetes, congestive heart failure, or blood clotting problems Severe pain	**Refer for treatment within minutes** Notify physician Administer O_2 per facility protocol EKG per facility protocol IV per facility protocol Administer aspirin per facility protocol Administer nitroglycerin per facility protocol Many diagnostic studies or procedures Frequent consultation Continuous monitoring If chest pain severe and worsens with breathing, movement, palpitation, or coughing, consider Level 3

Acuity Level/Assessment	Nursing Considerations
Level 3: Moderate Risk	**Urgent**
Moderate pain Stable vital signs and rhythm Age <35 yr and heart palpitations No difficulty breathing Heavy smoker Pain, swelling, warmth, or redness of leg Pain with exertion Strong family history of heart disease, heart attack, stroke, or diabetes	**Refer for treatment as soon as possible** Monitor for changes in condition May need multiple diagnostic studies or procedures If abnormal vital signs, consider Level 2
Level 4: Low Risk	**Semi-Urgent**
Recent injury and pain increases with movement and inspiration Fever, cough, congestion	Reassess while waiting, per facility protocol Offer comfort measures May need simple diagnostic study or procedure
Level 5: Lower Risk	Non-Urgent
Pain worsens when pressure applied to the area Intermittent pain increases with deep breathing and coughing Chronic pain	Reassess while waiting, per facility protocol Offer comfort measures May need examination only

RELATED PROTOCOLS:

Breathing Problems • Cold Symptoms

See Appendix H: Differential Diagnosis of Chest Pain

Cold Exposure, Hypothermia/Frostbite

KEY QUESTIONS:
Name • Age • Onset • Length and Time of Exposure • Body Temperature • Vital Signs
• Pain Scale • Medications • Tetanus Status

Acuity Level/Assessment	Nursing Considerations
Level 1: Critical	**Resuscitation**
Apnea or severe respiratory distress Pulseless Unresponsive	**Immediate treatment** Staff at bedside Mobilization of resuscitation team Many resources needed
Level 2: High Risk	**Emergent**
Altered mental status lethargy Depressed level of consciousness Muscle rigidity Skin hard, cold, white, blue, yellow, or waxy (3rd-degree frostbite) Purple fingers, toes, or nail beds Unable to raise body temperature Poor coordination or lightheadedness Infant, elderly, disabled, or immunosuppressed	**Do not delay treatment** Notify physician Multiple diagnostic studies or procedures Frequent consultation Continuous monitoring Re-warm as soon as possible
Level 3: Moderate Risk	**Urgent**
Severe pain Blistering or peeling skin (2nd-degree frostbite) Persistent shivering after warming	**Refer for treatment as soon as possible** Monitor for changes in condition May need multiple diagnostic studies or procedures If abnormal vital signs, consider Level 2
Level 4: Low Risk	**Semi-Urgent**

Signs of infection (redness, swelling, pain, red
   streaks, warmth)
Cold, mild shivering
Redness followed by blister formation in 24 to
   36 hr and skin is soft
	Reassess while waiting, per facility protocol
	Offer comfort measures
	May need a simple diagnostic study or
	   procedure

Acuity Level/Assessment	Nursing Considerations
Level 5: Lower Risk	Non-Urgent
Cold but no skin blistering Able to talk and drink warm fluids Asymptomatic	Reassess while waiting, per facility protocol Offer comfort measures May need an examination only

Notes

Cold Symptoms

KEY QUESTIONS:
Name • Age • Onset • Allergies • Prior History • Associated Symptoms • Pain Scale • Vital Signs • Oxygen Saturation • Medications

Acuity Level/Assessment	Nursing Considerations
● ● ● Level 1: Critical	**Resuscitation**
Apnea or severe respiratory distress Pale, diaphoretic, and lightheaded or weak O_2 saturation <90% with oxygen	**Refer for immediate treatment** Many resources needed Staff at bedside Mobilization of resuscitation team
● ● ● Level 2: High Risk	**Emergent**
Altered mental status Difficulty breathing (unrelated to nasal congestion) Chest pain (unrelated to chest wall movement) Petechiae, fever, headache, pain with neck flexion O_2 saturation <94% with oxygen O_2 saturation <90% on room air Infant <12 wk old with a temperature >100.4°F (38.0°C)	**Do not delay treatment** Notify physician Multiple diagnostic studies or procedures Frequent consultation Constant monitoring
● ● ● Level 3: Moderate Risk	**Urgent**
Severe pain Fever >103°F (39.4°C) Child >12 wk old and fever >105°F (41.5°C) Signs of dehydration Neck pain or rigidity History of immunosuppression, >60 yr or diabetes, and fever >100.5°F (38.1°C) Chest pain with deep inspiration or coughing	**Refer for treatment as soon as possible** May need multiple diagnostic studies or procedures Monitor for changes in condition If vital signs abnormal, consider Level 2

Acuity Level/Assessment	Nursing Considerations
Level 4: Low Risk	**Semi-Urgent**
Moderate pain Intermittent wheezing unrelated to diagnosed asthma History of chronic illness Sinus pain, sore throat, or fever persists >3 days Green or brown sputum >72 hr	Reassess while waiting, per facility protocol Offer comfort measures May need a simple diagnostic study or procedure
Level 5: Lower Risk	Non-Urgent
Earache Sore throat Runny nose Intermittent cough	Reassess while waiting, per facility protocol Offer comfort measures May need examination only

RELATED PROTOCOLS:

Breathing Problems • Fever • Sore Throat

Notes

Confusion

Acuity Level/Assessment	Nursing Considerations
●●● **Level 1: Critical**	**Resuscitation**
Apnea or severe difficulty breathing Pale, diaphoretic, lightheaded, or weak Status epilepticus Hypotension Unresponsive	**Immediate treatment** Staff at bedside Mobilization of resuscitation team Many resources needed
●●● **Level 2: High Risk**	**Emergent**
Recent head injury or trauma with loss of consciousness Drug or alcohol overdose Exposure to chemicals or ingestion of drug(s) Disoriented to name, date, or place Temperature >102°F (38.9°C) Headache, fever, and stiff or painful neck Sudden weakness on one side of the body Difficulty speaking	**Do not delay treatment** Notify physician Multiple diagnostic studies or procedures Frequent consultation Continuous monitoring
●●● **Level 3: Moderate Risk**	**Urgent**

History of psychosis
History of diabetes, stroke, high blood
  pressure, or cardiac disease
Fever >101°F (38.3°C) in the elderly or
  immunosuppressed
History of drug or alcohol abuse
	Refer for treatment as soon as possible
	Monitor for changes in condition
	May need multiple diagnostic studies or
	  procedures
	If abnormal vital signs, consider Level 2

Acuity Level/Assessment	Nursing Considerations
●●● **Level 4: Low Risk**	**Semi-Urgent**
Taking medications known to cause confusion Recently taking a new medication History of seizure disorder Persistent confusion after fever clears History of dementia or chronic brain syndrome and change in status Low-grade fever	Reassess while waiting, per facility protocol Offer comfort measures May need a simple diagnostic study or procedure
●●● Level 5: Lower Risk	Non-Urgent
History of dementia or chronic brain syndrome and no change in status Afebrile	Reassess while waiting, per facility protocol Offer comfort measures May need an examination only

RELATED PROTOCOLS:
Altered Mental Status • Fever

Notes

Contusion

?

KEY QUESTIONS:
Name • Age • Onset • Allergies • Prior History • Severity • Pain Scale • Vital Signs • Oxygen Saturation • Specifics of Injury • Medications

Acuity Level/Assessment	Nursing Considerations
●●● **Level 1: Critical**	**Resuscitation**
Apnea or severe respiratory distress Pulseless Unresponsive Pale, diaphoretic, and lightheaded or weak	**Refer for immediate treatment** Staff at bedside Mobilization of resuscitation team Many resources needed
●●● **Level 2: High Risk**	**Emergent**
Altered mental status Chest pain Blunt chest or abdominal trauma Chest, flank, or abdominal wall bruising Possibility of deep trauma (solid organ laceration, hollow organ rupture) Risk of domestic violence (separate patient from visitor for safety) History inconsistent with injuries Battle sign or raccoon eyes Circumferential ecchymoses of neck Fever, weakness, tachycardia, hypotension	**Do not delay treatment** Notify physician Multiple diagnostic studies or procedures Frequent consultation Continuous monitoring Refer to Bruise Assessment chart to determine age of contusion (page 50)
●●● **Level 3: Moderate Risk**	**Urgent**
Severe pain Trauma and possibility of a fracture or muscle hematoma Bite marks Bruising over multiple areas Difficulty walking	**Refer for treatment as soon as possible** May need multiple diagnostic studies or procedures Monitor for changes in condition Monitor circulation, movement, and sensation of affected extremity

Acuity Level/Assessment	Nursing Considerations
Level 3: Moderate Risk	**Urgent**
History of bleeding problems or use of blood thinners Increased pain, swelling, redness, fever, or red streaks	Refer to Bruise Assessment chart below to determine age of contusion If vital signs abnormal, consider Level 2
Level 4: Low Risk	**Semi-Urgent**
Moderate pain Small bruises on extremities	Reassess while waiting, per facility protocol Offer comfort measure May need simple diagnostic study or procedure Refer to Bruise Assessment chart below to determine age of contusion
Level 5: Lower Risk	Non-Urgent
Contusion healing but patient or parent concerned No other symptoms	Reassess while waiting, per facility protocol Offer comfort measures May need examination only Refer to Bruise Assessment chart below to determine age of contusion

RELATED PROTOCOLS:

Extremity Injury

Bruise Assessment	
Color of Bruise	**Age of Bruise**
Red, reddish blue	Less than 24 hr since time of injury
Dark blue, dark purple	1 to 4 days
Green, yellow-green	5 to 7 days
Yellow, brown	7 to 10 days
Normal tint, disappearance of bruise	1 to 3 wk

Cough

KEY QUESTIONS:

Name • Age • Onset • Allergies • Prior History • Severity • Pain Scale • Vital Signs • Oxygen Saturation • Medications • Associated Symptoms

Acuity Level/Assessment	Nursing Considerations
●●● **Level 1: Critical**	**Resuscitation**
Apnea or severe respiratory distress Unresponsive Unable to speak Oxygen saturation <90% with oxygen Central cyanosis	**Immediate treatment** Staff at bedside Mobilization of resuscitation team Many resources needed
●●● **Level 2: High Risk**	**Emergent**
Altered mental status Drooling Severe difficulty breathing Intercostal and substernal retractions Severe stridor Speaking in short words Blue lips or tongue Feeling of suffocation Frothy pink sputum Child <12 mo with rapid breathing and persistent cough	**Do not delay treatment** Notify physician Multiple diagnostic studies or procedures Frequent consultation Continuous monitoring
●●● **Level 3: Moderate Risk**	**Urgent**
Severe pain Speaking in partial sentences Mild stridor Wheezing heard across the room History of asthma and non-responsive to home care Fever >103°F (39.4°C) Fever >100.5°F (38.1°C) and age >60 yr or immunosuppressed	**Refer for treatment as soon as possible** Monitor for changes in condition May need multiple diagnostic studies or procedures If abnormal vital signs, consider Level 2

Acuity Level/Assessment	Nursing Considerations
Level 3: Moderate Risk	**Urgent**
Coughing up blood Cough unrelated to cold symptoms and history of recent trauma, surgery, childbirth, heart attacks, blood clots, or long sedentary period	
Level 4: Low Risk	**Semi-Urgent**
Moderate pain Speaking in full sentences No stridor Occus wheezing, rales, or rhonchi with auscultation History of asthma and has not taken medication or a breathing treatment Persistent fever >72 hr and no response to fever-reducing measures Coughing interferes with sleep Intermittent barking cough unrelieved by exposure to cool air, humidifier, or steam Green or brown sputum >72 hr	Reassess while waiting, per facility protocol Offer comfort measures May need a simple diagnostic study or procedure
Level 5: Lower Risk	Non-Urgent
History of croup Cough caused by exercise Intermittent chest discomfort with deep, productive coughing No other signs or symptoms but parent or patient concerned Cough and weight loss Earache Sore throat	Reassess while waiting, per facility protocol Offer comfort measures May need an examination only

RELATED PROTOCOLS:
Asthma • Breathing Problems • Cold Symptoms

Crying Baby

Name • Age • Onset • Allergies • Prior History (Including Birth History) • Severity • Pain Scale • Vital Signs • Oxygen Saturation

Acuity Level/Assessment	Nursing Considerations
Level 1: Critical	**Resuscitation**
Apnea or severe respiratory distress Central cyanosis	**Immediate treatment** Staff at bedside Mobilization of resuscitation team Many resources needed
Level 2: High Risk	**Emergent**
Altered mental status Temperature >100.4°F (38°C) in infants <12 wk Blue lips or tongue Petechiae Extreme lethargy	**Do not delay treatment** Notify physician Multiple diagnostic studies or procedures Frequent consultation Continuous monitoring
Level 3: Moderate Risk	**Urgent**

Inability to console infant
Recent trauma
Risk of abuse
Unexplained bruising
Intermittent lethargy or irritability
Persistent crying >2 hr
Projectile vomiting
	Refer for treatment as soon as possible
	Monitor for change in condition
	May need multiple diagnostic studies or
	   procedures
	If abnormal vital signs, consider Level 2
	If suspected abuse, keep infant under
	   observation

Level 4: Low Risk	**Semi-Urgent**
Recent use of "cold" medication Fever, vomiting, cold symptoms Raised, red, or itchy rash Fever, vomiting, or pulling ears	Reassess while waiting, per facility protocol Offer comfort measures May need a simple diagnostic study or procedure

Acuity Level/Assessment	Nursing Considerations
Level 5: Lower Risk	Non-Urgent
>2 hr since last feeding >3 hr since last nap Recent immunizations and fever	Reassess while waiting, per facility protocol Offer comfort measures May need an examination only

Notes

Depression

KEY QUESTIONS:
Name • Age • Onset • Allergies • Prior History • Severity • Pain Scale • Vital Signs
• Medications

Acuity Level/Assessment	Nursing Considerations
Level 1: Critical	**Resuscitation**
Severe respiratory distress Hypotension Pale, diaphoretic, and lightheaded or weak	**Immediate treatment** Staff at bedside Mobilization of resuscitation team Many resources needed
Level 2: High Risk	**Emergent**
Altered mental status Suicidal or homicidal gesture Overdose or other potentially serious attempt at self-harm Psychosis	**Do not delay treatment** Notify physician Multiple diagnostic studies or procedures Frequent consultation Continuous monitoring
Level 3: Moderate Risk	**Urgent**

Severe pain
Suicidal/homicidal ideation with a plan and
    the means to carry out the plan
Past inpatient psychiatric admission for
    depression
Adolescent acting out, provocative or risk-
    taking behavior
Recent childbirth, family loss, trauma, or
    emotional trauma
Change in behavior, crying, or withdrawal
Anxiety interferes with daily activity
	Refer for treatment as soon as possible
	Monitor for changes in condition
	May need multiple diagnostic studies or
	    procedures
	If abnormal vital signs, consider Level 2
	Keep suicidal patient under observation while
	    waiting to be seen
	Contact crisis or social worker, per facility
	    protocol

Level 4: Low Risk	**Semi-Urgent**
Moderate pain Suicidal thoughts without a plan or the means to carry out the plan	Reassess while waiting, per facility protocol Offer comfort measures

Acuity Level/Assessment	Nursing Considerations
Level 4: Low Risk	**Semi-Urgent**
Difficulty concentrating, sleeping, or maintaining interpersonal relationships Inability to experience pleasure Ethyl alcohol ingestion Situational depression Change in medication or dose Out of medication	May need a simple diagnostic study or procedure
Level 5: Lower Risk	Non-Urgent
Reported history of depression with no current signs or symptoms	Reassess while waiting, per facility protocol Offer comfort measures May need an examination only

RELATED PROTOCOLS:

Anxiety

Notes

Diabetic Problems

Name • Age • Onset • Allergies • Prior History • Severity • Pain Scale • Vital Signs • Oxygen Saturation • Serum Glucose Level • Medications

Acuity Level/Assessment	Nursing Considerations
●●● **Level 1: Critical**	**Resuscitation**
Apnea or severe respiratory distress Hypotension Unresponsive Pale, diaphoretic, and lightheaded or weak Seizure	**Refer for immediate treatment** Many resources needed Staff at bedside Mobilization of resuscitation team
●●● **Level 2: High Risk**	**Emergent**
Altered mental status Intractable vomiting Blood sugar <60 Hypoglycemic infant Insulin overdose	**Do not delay treatment** Notify physician Multiple diagnostic studies or procedures Frequent consultation Constant monitoring Measure serum glucose level
●●● **Level 3: Moderate Risk**	**Urgent**
Severe pain Blood sugar >400 or < 80 Rapid respiratory rate Fruity breath odor Lightheaded Profuse diaphoresis Wound with signs of infection: drainage, fever, red streaks, or pus Persistent vomiting and inability to keep down medication	**Refer for treatment as soon as possible** May need multiple diagnostic studies or procedures Monitor for changes in condition If vital signs abnormal, consider Level 2 Measure serum glucose level
●●● **Level 4: Low Risk**	**Semi-Urgent**
Moderate pain Slow healing wound	Reassess while waiting, per facility protocol Offer comfort measures

Acuity Level/Assessment	Nursing Considerations
Level 4: Low Risk	**Semi-Urgent**
Upper respiratory infection with fever and cough Headache or nausea and prolonged period since last meal	May need a simple diagnostic study or procedure
Level 5: Lower Risk	Non-Urgent
Request for prescription refill New-onset insulin-dependent diabetes mellitus and requests additional education for self-administration of insulin	Reassess while waiting, per facility protocol Offer comfort measures May need examination only

RELATED PROTOCOLS:
Altered Mental Status • Fever • Wound Infection

Notes

Diarrhea, Adult

KEY QUESTIONS:
Name • Age • Onset • Allergies • Prior History • Severity of Symptoms • Pain Scale
• Vital Signs • Medications • Diet • Travel • Family Members • Laxatives • Chronic Diarrhea
• Abdominal Surgery • Recent Antibiotic Therapy • Drinking from Wells or Streams

Acuity Level/Assessment	Nursing Considerations
Level 1: Critical	**Resuscitation**
Unresponsive Apnea or severe respiratory distress	**Immediate treatment** Many resources needed Staff at bedside Mobilization of resuscitation team
Level 2: High Risk	**Emergent**
Confusion, lethargy, disorientation Altered mental status Severe weakness or lightheadedness Pallor, diaphoresis Large amounts frank bloody stool	**Do not delay treatment** Notify physician Multiple diagnostic studies or procedures Frequent consultation Continuous monitoring
Level 3: Moderate Risk	**Urgent**
Severe abdominal pain >2 hr Signs of dehydration: decreased urination, sunken eyes, loose dry skin, excessive thirst, dry mouth Lightheadedness upon standing Fever >101°F (38.3°C) and unresponsive to fever-reducing measures Diarrhea every 30 to 60 min for >6 hr Diarrhea >5 days Loss of bowel control Persistent vomiting >3 days	**Refer for treatment as soon as possible** Monitor for changes in condition May need multiple diagnostic studies or procedures Collect/save stool specimen, per facility protocol If vital signs abnormal, consider Level 2 If tolerating oral fluids, give small amounts frequently

Acuity Level/Assessment	Nursing Considerations
Level 4: Low Risk	**Semi-Urgent**
Yellow, green, or frothy stool Moderate abdominal pain Diarrhea >6 times/24 hr Diarrhea >2 days Low-grade fever Nausea	Reassess while waiting, per facility protocol Offer comfort measures May need simple diagnostic study or procedure
Level 5: Lower Risk	Non-Urgent
Diarrhea <6 times/24 hr Loose stools	Reassess while waiting, per facility protocol Offer comfort measures May need examination only

RELATED PROTOCOLS:

Abdominal Pain, Adult • Poisoning, Exposure or Ingestion • Vomiting

Notes

Diarrhea, Pediatric

Acuity Level/Assessment	Nursing Considerations
●●● **Level 1: Critical**	**Resuscitation**
Unresponsive Apnea or severe respiratory distress Pale, diaphoretic, and lightheaded or weak Hypotensive	**Immediate treatment** Many resources needed Staff at bedside Mobilization of resuscitation team
●●● **Level 2: High Risk**	**Emergent**
Confusion, lethargy, disorientation Altered mental status Severe weakness or lightheadedness Cold, gray skin Large amounts frank bloody stool Infant <12 wks and fever >100.4°F (38.0°C) Capillary refill >2 seconds	**Do not delay treatment** Notify physician Multiple diagnostic studies or procedures Frequent consultation Constant monitoring
●●● **Level 3: Moderate Risk**	**Urgent**
Signs of dehydration: age <1 yr and no urine >8 hr, age >1 yr and no urine >12 hr, sunken eyes or fontanels, crying without tears, excessive thirst, dry mouth Severe abdominal pain (drawing knees to chest with cramping) Lightheadedness upon standing Fever >105°F (40.6°C) and unresponsive to fever-reducing measures >3 months old Age <1 mo and diarrhea >3 times Age <1 yr and diarrhea >8 times/8 hr	**Refer for treatment as soon as possible** Reassess, per facility protocol Monitor for changes in condition May need multiple diagnostic studies or procedures Collect/save stool specimen, per facility protocol If vital signs abnormal, consider Level 2 If tolerating oral fluids, give small amounts frequently

Acuity Level/Assessment	Nursing Considerations
Level 3: Moderate Risk	**Urgent**
Abdominal pain >2 hr and no improvement with each episode of diarrhea Vomiting clear fluids and watery diarrhea >3 times	
Level 4: Low Risk	**Semi-Urgent**
Diarrhea >3 days Fever unresponsive to fever-reducing measures Temperature >103°F (39.4°C) Temperature >101°F (38.3°C) > 24 hr Bloody stools Receiving antibiotic therapy	Reassess while waiting, per facility protocol Offer comfort measures May need simple diagnostic study or procedure
Level 5: Lower Risk	Non-Urgent
Chronic diarrhea Recent diet change Bloody stools and history of anal fissure	Reassess while waiting, per facility protocol Offer comfort measures May need examination only

RELATED PROTOCOLS:

Abdominal Pain, Pediatric • Poisoning, Exposure or Ingestion • Vomiting

Notes

Ear Problems
(for foreign body, see Foreign Body, Ear)

KEY QUESTIONS:
Name • Age • Onset • History • Temperature • Allergies • Medication • Pain Scale
• Vital Signs

Acuity Level/Assessment	Nursing Considerations
Level 1: Critical	**Resuscitation**
Severe respiratory distress Pale, diaphoretic, and lightheaded or weak	**Immediate treatment** Staff at bedside Mobilization of resuscitation team Many resources needed
Level 2: High Risk	**Emergent**
Confusion, lethargy, disorientation Altered mental status Injury and fluid leaking from ear Battle sign (bruising behind ear) with head trauma	**Do not delay treatment** Notify physician Multiple diagnostic studies or procedures Frequent consultation Continuous monitoring Check for CSF with head trauma
Level 3: Moderate Risk	**Urgent**
Severe pain Pain, swelling, and bloody and/or purulent discharge from ear Redness or facial drooping on affected side of face associated with blow to head Sudden hearing loss with pain Pain unresponsive to analgesics History of diabetes/immunosuppression and earpain	**Refer for treatment as soon as possible** Monitor for changes in condition May need multiple diagnostic studies or procedures If abnormal vital signs, consider Level 2

Acuity Level/Assessment	Nursing Considerations
Level 4: Low Risk	**Semi-Urgent**
Mild tenderness on bone behind ear Slight swelling, pain, warmth, drainage, low-grade fever Unable to remove wax plug with medication Decreased hearing, along with pain with cracking or popping noise Mild/intermittent ringing in ears Antibiotics for ear infection >3 days and earache persists	Reassess while waiting, per facility protocol Offer comfort measures May need a simple diagnostic study or procedure Do not instill liquid drops if eardrum rupture suspected
Level 5: Lower Risk	Non-Urgent
Sunburn Itching Pain after exposure to cold Pain after swimming or exposure to water	Reassess while waiting, per facility protocol Offer comfort measures May need an examination only

RELATED PROTOCOLS:

Foreign Body, Ear

Notes

Electric Shock/Lightning Injury

KEY QUESTIONS:
Name • Age • Onset • Cause • Vital Signs • Pain Scale • Entrance and Exit Wounds • Oxygen Saturation

Acuity Level/Assessment	Nursing Considerations
Level 1: Critical	**Resuscitation**
Apnea or severe respiratory distress Pulseless Unresponsive Pale, diaphoretic, and lightheaded or weak Hypotension	**Refer for immediate treatment** Staff at bedside Mobilization of resuscitation team Many resources needed
Level 2: High Risk	**Emergent**
Confusion, lethargy, disorientation Severe pain Altered mental status Weakness, chest pain, irregular pulse, palpitations Evidence of burn marks (entrance and/or exit wounds) Seizure Age <18 mo History of unconsciousness Pallor, diaphoresis Oxygen saturation <92%	**Do not delay treatment** Notify physician Multiple diagnostic studies or procedures Frequent consultation Continuous monitoring Monitor for internal injury, even if no external signs of burn are present Perform frequent extremity vascular checks Obtain 12-lead EKG as soon as possible Observe for entrance/exit burn wounds Start IV if patient burned or monitoring shows abnormalities
Level 3: Moderate Risk	**Urgent**
History of cardiac disease Exposure to 220-W voltage or greater Burn to face Bloody/cloudy urine	**Refer for treatment as soon as possible** Monitor for changes in condition Monitor for internal injury, even with no external signs of burn Perform frequent extremity vascular checks May need multiple diagnostic studies or procedures

Acuity Level/Assessment	Nursing Considerations
Level 3: Moderate Risk	**Urgent**
Muscle pain Headache Fatigue	Obtain 12-lead EKG as soon as possible Apply dry dressing to burn wounds If abnormal vital signs, consider Level 2
Level 4: Low Risk	**Semi-Urgent**
Asymptomatic but parent or patient concerned	Reassess while waiting, per facility protocol Offer comfort measures May need simple diagnostic study or procedure
Level 5: Lower Risk	Non-Urgent
	Reassess while waiting, per facility protocol Offer comfort measures May need an examination only

RELATED PROTOCOLS:
Chest Pain • Extremity Injury

Notes

Extremity Injury

KEY QUESTIONS:

Name • Age • Onset • Allergies • Prior History • Severity • Pain Scale • Cause • Vital Signs • Oxygen Saturation • Neurovascular Status of Extremity

Acuity Level/Assessment	Nursing Considerations
●●● **Level 1: Critical**	**Resuscitation**
Apnea or severe difficulty breathing Unresponsive Pulseless Pale, diaphoretic, and lightheaded or weak Pulsatile bleeding	**Refer for immediate treatment** Staff at bedside Mobilization of resuscitation team Many resources needed Apply pressure dressing to stop bleeding
●●● **Level 2: High Risk**	**Emergent**
Altered mental status Severe pain in hip or thigh after traumatic injury and unable to ambulate Bone protrudes through the skin Partial or complete amputation Penetrating wound and object still present Unable to stop bleeding with pressure Fingers or toes of affected limb are cold, pale, mottled or numb No pulse in affected extremity and cyanosis/pallor Prolonged capillary refill >2–3 seconds High-pressure injection injury	**Do not delay treatment** Notify physician Multiple diagnostic studies or procedures Frequent consultation Continuous monitoring Do not remove penetrating object Apply pressure dressing to stop bleeding
●●● **Level 3: Moderate Risk**	**Urgent**
Deformed limb Severe pain with movement or weight bearing Unable to move part of arm, hand, or foot distal to deep laceration Unable to remove ring and distal digit is turning pale, white, or blue Severe swelling, pain, and loss of sensation	**Refer for treatment as soon as possible** May need multiple diagnostic studies or procedures Monitor for changes in condition If vital signs abnormal, consider Level 2 Remove ring from swollen digit Apply splint, per facility protocol

Acuity Level/Assessment	Nursing Considerations
Level 3: Moderate Risk	**Urgent**
Increasing swelling or bruising around wound of person taking anticoagulants Puncture wound into a joint Numbness and tingling Open fracture Fever, drainage, red streaks	Elevate and apply ice pack for pain or swelling Assess ankle injury using Ottawa criteria Order radiographs, per facility protocol
Level 4: Low Risk	**Semi-Urgent**
Pain with movement or weight bearing Difficulty moving the joint nearest the injury Puncture wound through sole of shoe Reported pop or snap at time of injury Suspicious history of injury (suspect abuse) Visible debris in wound after scrubbing History of diabetes No improvement in pain >3 days post injury Numbness or tingling	Offer comfort measures Reassess while waiting, per facility protocol May need simple diagnostic study or procedure Remove ring from swollen digit Apply splint, per facility protocol Elevate and apply ice pack for pain or swelling Assess ankle injury using Ottawa criteria Order radiographs, per facility protocol
Level 5: Lower Risk	Non-Urgent
Pain, swelling, or discoloration Chronic discomfort with old injury History of arthritis or tendonitis No improvement in swelling >2 wk post injury	Offer comfort measures Reassess while waiting, per facility protocol May need examination only

RELATED PROTOCOLS:
Electrical Shock • Laceration • Puncture Wound

Eye Injury or Problems

KEY QUESTIONS:
Name • Age • Onset • Cause • Allergies • Corrective Glasses or Contact Use • Visual Acuity • Vital Signs • Tetanus Immunization Status • Medications

Acuity Level/Assessment	Nursing Considerations
●●● Level 1: Critical	**Resuscitation**
Apnea or severe respiratory distress Pulseless Unresponsive	**Immediate treatment** Staff at bedside Mobilization of resuscitation team Many resources needed
●●● Level 2: High Risk	**Emergent**
Altered mental status Laceration or penetrating injury to eye Blow or trauma to eye with marked loss of vision Flashing light in visual field Blood in iris (colored part of eye) Clear, jelly-like discharge from injured eye Corneal burn (exposure of eye to alkali or acid) Unilateral painless loss of vision	**Do not delay treatment** Notify physician Multiple diagnostic studies or procedures Frequent consultation Continuous monitoring Immediate irrigation for chemical burns Instill optic anesthetic, per facility protocol Consider c-spine injury with traumatic injury
●●● Level 3: Moderate Risk	**Urgent**
Severe pain Burn to eye (thermal or light) Persistent blurred/double vision Swelling, pain, tearing of eye Eye pain associated with facial/orbital trauma Ecchymosis surrounding eye Increasing pain with eye movement Laceration to eyelid Foreign body in eye Swollen eyelids red, warm to touch, and fever > 101.4	**Refer for treatment as soon as possible** Monitor for changes in condition May need multiple diagnostic studies or procedures Offer cool compresses to reduce swelling Instill optic anesthetic, per facility protocol If vital signs abnormal, consider Level 2

Acuity Level/Assessment	Nursing Considerations
Level 4: Low Risk	**Semi-Urgent**
Discomfort or irritation persists 24 hr after injury or removal of foreign body Signs of infection develop after injury: mild pain, swelling, redness, drainage, or fever Small blood vessel rupture in sclera Fever < 101.4 and swollen red eyelids or tear duct Persistent itching, redness, burning, and discharge History of improper contact lens usage; inability to remove contacts	Reassess while waiting, per facility protocol Offer comfort measures May need a simple diagnostic study or procedure
Level 5: Lower Risk	Non-Urgent
Dry eyes and itching Mild eye crusting Asymptomatic	Reassess while waiting, per facility protocol Offer comfort measures May need an examination only

Notes

Feeding Tube Problems

Name • Age • Prior History • Onset • Type of Tube • Length of Time Tube in Place • Pain Scale • Vital Signs

Acuity Level/Assessment	Nursing Considerations
●●● **Level 1: Critical**	**Resuscitation**
Apnea or severe respiratory distress Unresponsive Pale, diaphoretic, and lightheaded or weak	**Immediate treatment** Staff at bedside Mobilization of resuscitation team Many resources needed
●●● **Level 2: High Risk**	**Emergent**
Altered mental status Severe bleeding through or at site of tube	**Do not delay treatment** Notify physician Multiple diagnostic studies or procedures Frequent consultation Continuous monitoring
●●● **Level 3: Moderate Risk**	**Urgent**
Severe pain Swelling, bleeding, or foul-smelling purulent discharge at insertion site	**Refer for treatment as soon as possible** Monitor for change in condition May need multiple diagnostic studies or procedures If vital signs abnormal, consider Level 2
●●● Level 4: Low Risk	Semi-Urgent
Moderate pain Signs of infection at insertion site: mild redness, swelling, pain, red streaks, or drainage Feeding tube dislodged or fallen out	Reassess while waiting, per facility protocol Offer comfort measures May need a simple diagnostic study or procedure

Acuity Level/Assessment	Nursing Considerations
Level 5: Lower Risk	Non-Urgent
Tube frequently clogs after feeding or medication administration Unable to unclog after trying home care measures Possible tube displacement Unable to pass solution into feeding tube Asymptomatic	Reassess while waiting, per facility protocol Offer comfort measures May need an examination only

Notes

Fever

Acuity Level/Assessment	Nursing Considerations
●●● **Level 1: Critical**	**Resuscitation**
Apnea or severe respiratory distress Unresponsive Pale, diaphoretic, and lightheaded or weak	**Immediate treatment** Staff at bedside Mobilization of resuscitation team Many resources needed
●●● **Level 2: High Risk**	**Emergent**
Confusion or disorientation Altered mental status Excessive drooling or difficulty swallowing Age <12 wk and temperature >100.4°F (38.0°C) Lethargy Petechiae Severe signs of dehydration in elderly, pediatric, immunosuppressed, or compromised patient Anuria or decreased urine output >24 hr Sunken eyes or fontanel, poor skin turgor, or excessive thirst in infant Severe headache, neck stiffness, neck pain, and photophobia	**Do not delay treatment** Notify physician Multiple diagnostic studies or procedures Frequent consultation Continuous monitoring
●●● **Level 3: Moderate Risk**	**Urgent**
Severe pain Temperature >104°F (40°C) and unresponsive to fever-reducing measures Temperature >102°F (39°C) and: Flank or back pain and painful/bloody urination	**Refer for treatment as soon as possible** Monitor for change in condition May need multiple diagnostic studies or procedures If vital signs abnormal, consider Level 2

Acuity Level/Assessment	Nursing Considerations
Level 3: Moderate Risk	**Urgent**
Shortness of breath, pleuritic pain, wheezing and/or productive cough History of diabetes, cancer, HIV/AIDS, kidney/liver disease, pregnancy, or recent surgery Nausea/vomiting Pediatric: Persistent irritability, inconsolable Infant age 3 to 6 mo and rectal temperature >102°F (39°C) with diarrhea, vomiting, and dehydration	Administer acetaminophen or ibuprofen, per facility protocol
Level 4: Low Risk	**Semi-Urgent**
Low-grade fever persists >72 hr and no known cause Earache, sore throat, mildly swollen glands Rash Frequent and/or mild burning with urination Vaginal discharge	Reassess while waiting, per facility protocol Offer comfort measures May need a simple diagnostic study or procedure
Level 5: Lower Risk	Non-Urgent
Temp <101°F (38.2°C) with no other symptoms Recent immunization	Reassess while waiting, per facility protocol Offer comfort measures May need an examination only

Finger and Toe Problems

KEY QUESTIONS:
Name • Age • Onset • Allergies • Prior History • Severity • Pain Scale • Vital Signs • Medications

Acuity Level/Assessment	Nursing Considerations
Level 1: Critical	**Resuscitation**
Apnea or severe respiratory distress Pulseless Unresponsive	**Refer for immediate treatment** Staff at bedside Mobilization of resuscitation team Many resources needed
Level 2: High Risk	**Emergent**
Altered mental status Open fracture Amputation Digits are cold, pale, blue, or mottled and numb	**Do not delay treatment** Notify physician Multiple diagnostic studies or procedures Frequent consultation Continuous monitoring
Level 3: Moderate Risk	**Urgent**
Severe pain Prolonged capillary refill Obvious deformity with compromised circulation Crush trauma Unable to stop bleeding with pressure Puncture wound into a joint Inability to remove rings, and digit is turning blue, pale, or white Fever, drainage, warm to touch, red streaks Exposed or injured nail bed	**Refer for treatment as soon as possible** May need multiple diagnostic studies or procedures Monitor for change in condition Check capillary refill Monitor circulation, movement, and sensation of affected extremity If vital signs abnormal, consider Level 2
Level 4: Low Risk	**Semi-Urgent**
Moderate pain Swelling Decreased range of motion	Reassess while waiting, per facility protocol Offer comfort measures

Acuity Level/Assessment	Nursing Considerations
Level 4: Low Risk	**Semi-Urgent**

Bruising of the digit
Subungual hematoma
Pain and swelling at second
    metatarsophalangeal joint
Numbness or tingling
	May need simple diagnostic study or
	    procedure

Level 5: Lower Risk	Non-Urgent
Pain or swelling without injury Minor bleeding under the nail Digit pain and history of arthritis or old injury	Reassess while waiting, per facility protocol Offer comfort measures May need examination only

RELATED PROTOCOLS:
Extremity Injury

Notes

Foreign Body, Ear

Name • Age • Onset • Identification of Foreign Body • Prior History • Medications • Allergies • Pain Scale • Vital Signs

Acuity Level/Assessment	Nursing Considerations
●●● Level 1: Critical	**Resuscitation**
Severe respiratory distress Unresponsive Pale, diaphoretic, and lightheaded or weak	**Immediate treatment** Staff at bedside Mobilization of resuscitation team Many resources needed
●●● Level 2: High Risk	**Emergent**
Altered mental status Foreign body movement in ear causing hysteria (insect) Object impaled in ear CSF leaking from ear	**Do not delay treatment** Notify physician Multiple diagnostic studies or procedures Frequent consultation Continuous monitoring
●●● Level 3: Moderate Risk	**Urgent**
Severe pain Unable to remove foreign body Facial drooping on side of injury Loss of coordination	**Refer for treatment as soon as possible** Monitor for change in condition May need multiple diagnostic studies or procedures If abnormal vital signs, consider Level 2
●●● Level 4: Low Risk	**Semi-Urgent**
Foreign body in ear requiring simple removal Persistent discomfort Hearing loss Persistent bleeding >30 min Lacerated earlobe Severe swelling of earlobe External ear red and swollen	Reassess while waiting, per facility protocol Offer comfort measures May need a simple diagnostic study or procedure

Acuity Level/Assessment	Nursing Considerations
Level 5: Lower Risk	Non-Urgent
Foreign body removed but parent or patient concerned	Reassess while waiting, per facility protocol Offer comfort measures May need an examination only

RELATED PROTOCOLS:

Ear Problems • Laceration

Notes

Foreign Body, Ingested

KEY QUESTIONS:
Name • Age • Onset • Severity of Symptoms • Consideration for Poisoning • Foreign Object/Substance Ingested • Vital Signs • Medications

Acuity Level/Assessment	Nursing Considerations
●●● **Level 1: Critical**	**Resuscitation**
Apnea or severe respiratory distress Pulseless Unresponsive	**Refer for immediate treatment** Staff at bedside Mobilization of resuscitation team Many resources needed
●●● **Level 2: High Risk**	**Emergent**
Altered mental status Excessive salivation, drooling, or gagging Coughing, choking, or dyspnea Evidence of burn to lips and/or tongue Vomiting associated with possible corrosive substance Suicidal behavior Difficulty breathing Hematemesis Drooling Chest pain Poisonous substance	**Do not delay treatment** Notify physician Access poison control center as necessary (1-800-222-1222) Multiple diagnostic studies or procedures Frequent consultation Continual monitoring Observe suicidal patient until placed in a room
●●● **Level 3: Moderate Risk**	**Urgent**
Severe pain Nausea and vomiting Object ingested larger than a nickel in children Difficulty swallowing Sharp object Abdominal distention Object ingested larger than quarter in adult	**Refer for treatment as soon as possible** Engage family/emergency medical staff in identifying foreign object, if unknown Instruct parent/patient to check stool for object May need multiple diagnostic studies or procedures Monitor for change in condition If vital signs abnormal, consider Level 2

Acuity Level/Assessment	Nursing Considerations
Level 4: Low Risk	**Semi-Urgent**
Moderate pain Suspicious history or foreign body sensation	Offer comfort measures Reassess while waiting, per facility protocol May need simple diagnostic study or procedure
Level 5: Lower Risk	Non-Urgent
Small wood or plastic object or dull glass Object ingested smaller than a penny Asymptomatic but parent/patient is concerned	Offer comfort measures May need examination only Reassess while waiting, per facility protocol

RELATED PROTOCOLS:

Abdominal Pain, Adult • Abdominal Pain, Child • Foreign Body, Inhaled

Notes

Foreign Body, Inhaled

KEY QUESTIONS:

Name • Age • Onset • Allergies • Prior History • Severity of Symptoms • Pain Scale • Object Inhaled • Medications • Oxygen Saturation • Vital Signs

Acuity Level/Assessment	Nursing Considerations
Level 1: Critical	**Resuscitation**
Cyanosis Unresponsive Unable to speak O_2 saturation <90% with oxygen Pulseless Choking	**Immediate treatment** Staff at bedside Mobilization of resuscitation team Many resources needed
Level 2: High Risk	**Emergent**
Altered mental status Difficulty breathing Inspiratory stridor Bilateral wheezing Significant coughing Drooling Retractions Speaking in short words O_2 saturation <90% on room air O_2 saturation <94% with oxygen Pallor and diaphoresis Unequal breath sounds	**Do not delay treatment** Notify physician Multiple diagnostic studies or procedures Frequent consultation Continuous monitoring
Level 3: Moderate Risk	**Urgent**
Fever Severe pain Lightheadedness Unilateral wheezing Expiratory wheezing Nasal flaring Speaking in partial sentences	**Refer for treatment as soon as possible** Monitor for change in condition May need multiple diagnostic studies or procedures If abnormal vital signs, consider Level 2

Acuity Level/Assessment	Nursing Considerations
●●● **Level 4: Low Risk**	**Semi-Urgent**
Sensation of foreign body with no respiratory signs and symptoms Speaking in full sentences	Reassess while waiting, per facility protocol Offer comfort measures May need a simple diagnostic study or procedure
●●● Level 5: Lower Risk	Non-Urgent
No symptoms but parent or patient concerned O₂ saturation >95% on room air	Reassess while waiting, per facility protocol Offer comfort measures May need an examination only

RELATED PROTOCOLS:
Asthma • Breathing Problems • Foreign Body, Ingested

Notes

Foreign Body, Rectum or Vagina

KEY QUESTIONS:
Name • Age • Onset • Allergies • Prior History • Severity of Symptoms • Pain Scale • Vital Signs • Description of Object • Medications

Acuity Level/Assessment	Nursing Considerations
Level 1: Critical	**Resuscitation**
Unresponsive Pale, diaphoretic, and confused or weak Violent assault with weapon (e.g., knife, blunt object) Severe respiratory distress	**Immediate treatment** Many resources needed Staff at bedside Mobilization of resuscitation team
Level 2: High Risk	**Emergent**
Heavy rectal/vaginal bleeding Fever and systolic BP <100 Multiple injuries from assault Severe abdominal pain Altered mental status Traumatic injury to rectum or vagina with foreign object	**Do not delay treatment** Notify physician Multiple diagnostic studies or procedures Frequent consultation Constant monitoring
Level 3: Moderate Risk	**Urgent**
Urinary retention or hematuria Moderate rectal/vaginal bleeding Unable to remove foreign body High fever, chills, nausea, or vomiting Abdominal pain with movement Suspect sexual abuse Insertion of a sharp object	**Refer for treatment as soon as possible** Monitor for change in condition May need multiple diagnostic studies or procedures If vital signs abnormal, consider Level 2 If sexual abuse suspected and perpetrator present, move up to Level 2
Level 4: Low Risk	**Semi-Urgent**
Sensation of rectal or vaginal fullness Rectal/vaginal pain Peri-rectal abscess	Reassess while waiting, per facility protocol Offer comfort measures May need simple diagnostic study or procedure

Acuity Level/Assessment	Nursing Considerations
●●● **Level 4: Low Risk**	**Semi-Urgent**
Retained tampon or condom Scant rectal or vaginal bleeding Unable to pass stool	
●●● Level 5: Lower Risk	Non-Urgent
Report of possible foreign body and no signs or symptoms	Reassess while waiting, per facility protocol Offer comfort measures May need examination only

RELATED PROTOCOLS:
Rectal Problems • Sexual Assault • Vaginal Bleeding, Abnormal

Notes

Foreign Body, Skin

KEY QUESTIONS:
Name • Age • Onset • Allergies • Medications • Prior History • Severity • Pain Scale
• Vital Signs • Tetanus Status

Acuity Level/Assessment	Nursing Considerations
Level 1: Critical	**Resuscitation**
Unresponsive Apnea or severe respiratory distress Pale, diaphoretic, and confused or weak	**Refer for immediate treatment** Staff at bedside Mobilization of resuscitation team Many resources needed
Level 2: High Risk	**Emergent**
Febrile and abnormal vital signs (BP <100) Fish hook imbedded in the eye Heavy bleeding from injury site Altered mental status Object impaled and difficulty breathing	**Do not delay treatment** Notify physician Multiple diagnostic studies or procedures Frequent consultation Continuous monitoring
Level 3: Moderate Risk	**Urgent**
Object impaled in the face and no respiratory impairment Severe pain Object imbedded in a joint space Object deeply imbedded Obvious injury to tendons, nerves, or vessels High level of anxiety Substance adhered to facial area (e.g., eyelids)	**Refer for treatment as soon as possible** May need multiple diagnostic studies or procedures Monitor for change in condition Obtain radiograph(s) for metal foreign body, per facility protocol Do not soak area of foreign body If abnormal vital signs, consider Level 2
Level 4: Low Risk	**Semi-Urgent**
Non-removable fish hook Object imbedded with minimal bleeding or no loss of sensation or function Moderate pain	Offer comfort measures Reassess while waiting, per facility protocol May need simple diagnostic study or procedure

Acuity Level/Assessment	Nursing Considerations
Level 4: Low Risk	**Semi-Urgent**
Foreign substance adhered to skin (e.g., tar, super glue) Signs of infection: redness, fever, pain, red streaks, warmth, pus	
Level 5: Lower Risk	Non-Urgent
Minimal pain Pierced earring inside of an earlobe or other non-vital structure No symptoms but parent or person concerned	Offer comfort measures Reassess while waiting, per facility protocol May need examination only

RELATED PROTOCOLS:
Laceration • Wound Infection

Notes

Genital Problems, Male

Acuity Level/Assessment	Nursing Considerations
● ● ● Level 1: Critical	**Resuscitation**
Severe respiratory distress Pale, diaphoretic, and lightheaded or weak Hypotension Unresponsive	**Refer for immediate treatment** Staff at bedside Mobilization of resuscitation team Many resources needed
● ● ● Level 2: High Risk	**Emergent**
Altered mental status Trauma with heavy, pulsatile bleeding Sudden-onset unilateral testicular pain in patient <20 yr Priapism Foreign body in penis	**Do not delay treatment** Notify physician Multiple diagnostic studies or procedures Frequent consultation Continuous monitoring Do not remove penetrating object
● ● ● Level 3: Moderate Risk	**Urgent**
Blood at meatus Severe pain Fever and pain with urination Penis caught in zipper Severe swelling Urinary retention	**Refer for treatment as soon as possible** Monitor for change in condition May need multiple diagnostic studies or procedures If abnormal vital signs, consider Level 2
● ● ● Level 4: Low Risk	**Semi-Urgent**
Penile discharge with fever and pain Moderate pain Open sore or wound on penis Suspected sexually transmitted disease exposure Penile discharge Burning with urination	Reassess while waiting, per facility protocol Offer comfort measures May need simple diagnostic study or procedure

Acuity Level/Assessment	Nursing Considerations
Level 5: Lower Risk	Non-Urgent
Erectile dysfunction Pain during or after intercourse Loss of sexual interest	Reassess while waiting, per facility protocol Offer comfort measures May need an examination only

RELATED PROTOCOLS:
Urination Problems

Notes

Headache

KEY QUESTIONS:
Name • Age • Onset • Allergies • Medications • Prior History • Severity of Symptoms • Pain Scale • Vital Signs

Acuity Level/Assessment	Nursing Considerations
●●● **Level 1: Critical**	**Resuscitation**
Apnea or severe respiratory distress Pale, diaphoretic, and lightheaded or weak Pulseless Hypotension	**Immediate treatment** Staff at bedside Mobilization of resuscitation team Many resources needed
●●● **Level 2: High Risk**	**Emergent**
"Worst headache of my life" Fever and stiff or painful neck Sudden onset of unilateral weakness Altered mental status Difficulty speaking or swallowing Nuchal rigidity Hyperreflexia Petechia	**Do not delay treatment** Notify physician Multiple diagnostic studies or procedures Frequent consultation Continuous monitoring
●●● **Level 3: Moderate Risk**	**Urgent**
Acute onset of severe headache Vomiting/nausea Vision changes Exposure to chemicals or smoke Recent head injury/trauma Known exposure to meningitis (bacterial)	**Refer for treatment as soon as possible** Monitor for change in condition May need multiple diagnostic studies or procedures If vital signs abnormal, consider Level 2
●●● **Level 4: Low Risk**	**Semi-Urgent**
Low-grade fever History of migraines and photosensitivity Body aches Acute stress Fever	Reassess while waiting, per facility protocol Offer comfort measures May need a simple diagnostic study or procedure

Acuity Level/Assessment	Nursing Considerations
Level 5: Lower Risk	Non-Urgent
Sinus symptoms Cold symptoms Caffeine withdrawal Pain occurs with reading No other symptoms but parent or patient concerned	Reassess while waiting, per facility protocol Offer comfort measures May need an examination only

RELATED PROTOCOLS:
Cold Symptoms • Fever • Head Injury

See Appendix I: Headache: Common Characteristics

Notes

Head Injury

KEY QUESTIONS:

Name • Age • Onset • Allergies • Prior History • Severity of Symptoms • Pain Scale • Vital Signs • Oxygen Saturation • Medications • Glascow Coma Scale Score

Acuity Level/Assessment	Nursing Considerations
Level 1: Critical	**Resuscitation**
Unresponsive Seizure Apnea or severe respiratory distress Pale, diaphoretic, and lightheaded or weak Pulseless	**Immediate treatment** Staff at bedside Mobilization of resuscitation team Many resources needed
Level 2: High Risk	**Emergent**
Altered mental status Severe neck pain Uncontrolled bleeding High-risk mechanism of injury Clear drainage from nose or ears Change in speech New-onset weakness or numbness Battle sign or raccoon eyes Obvious dent to head	**Do not delay treatment** Notify physician Multiple diagnostic studies or procedures Frequent consultation Continuous monitoring Protect C-spine Refer to MVA Triage Questions (Appendix J)
Level 3: Moderate Risk	**Urgent**

History of loss of consciousness, fine now
Visual changes
Vomiting >3 times or projectile vomiting
Deceleration injury
Infant fall >2 ft
Suspect child abuse or neglect
Loss of memory, fine now
Change in balance or equilibrium
Facial lacerations
	Refer for treatment as soon as possible
	Monitor for changes in condition
	May need multiple diagnostic studies or
	    procedures
	If vital signs abnormal, consider Level 2
	Refer to Mechanisms of Injury
	    (Appendices K–N)
	Ice pack to help reduce swelling

Acuity Level/Assessment	Nursing Considerations
Level 4: Low Risk	**Semi-Urgent**
Nausea Infant fall <2 ft Injury and no loss of consciousness Headache >1 wk post injury	Reassess while waiting, per facility protocol Offer comfort measures May need a simple diagnostic study or procedure
Level 5: Lower Risk	Non-Urgent
No symptoms but parent or patient concerned	Reassess while waiting, per facility protocol Offer comfort measures May need an examination only

RELATED PROTOCOLS:

Headache • Motor Vehicle Accident

See Appendices J through N: MVA Triage Questions and Mechanisms of Injury

Notes

Heart Rate, Rapid

KEY QUESTIONS:

Name • Age • Onset • Allergies • Medications • Prior History • Severity of Symptoms • Pain Scale • Vital Signs • Oxygen Saturation • Cardiac History (stent, CABG, valve, MI, pacers)

Acuity Level/Assessment	Nursing Considerations
Level 1: Critical	**Resuscitation**
Apnea or severe respiratory distress Unresponsive Pale, diaphoretic, and lightheaded or weak Hypotension	**Refer for immediate treatment** Many resources needed Staff at bedside Mobilization of resuscitation team
Level 2: High Risk	**Emergent**
Altered mental status Chest, jaw, or arm pain Adult HR >150 Child HR >180 Difficulty breathing Facial cyanosis or pallor Possible overdose Lightheadedness or dizziness Unsteady walking Diaphoresis	**Do not delay treatment** Notify physician Multiple diagnostic studies or procedures Frequent consultation Continuous monitoring
Level 3: Moderate Risk	**Urgent**
History of heart disease, paroxysmal supraventricular tachycardia, or thyroid disease Intermittent episodes of fast heart rate History of antihistamine or diet pill use Signs of dehydration Possible drug ingestion or exposure Anxiety attact	**Refer for treatment as soon as possible** May need multiple diagnostic studies or procedures Monitor for change in condition If vital signs abnormal, consider Level 2

Acuity Level/Assessment	Nursing Considerations
Level 4: Low Risk	**Semi-Urgent**
Diarrhea Vomiting New medication Increased caffeine consumption Increased stress or emotional anxiety HR <140 and regular	Reassess while waiting, per facility protocol Offer comfort measures May need a simple diagnostic study or procedure
Level 5: Lower Risk	Non-Urgent
History of palpitations No symptoms Mild fever Associated pain or anxiety	Reassess while waiting, per facility protocol Offer comfort measures May need examination only

RELATED PROTOCOLS:

Anxiety • Breathing Problems • Chest Pain • Diarrhea, Adult • Diarrhea, Pediatric • Lightheadedness/Fainting • Vomiting

Notes

Heart Rate, Slow

Name • Age • Onset • Allergies • Medications • Prior History • Severity of Symptoms • Pain Scale • Vital Signs • Oxygen Saturation • Cardiac History (stent, CABG, pacer, MI)

Acuity Level/Assessment	Nursing Considerations
●●● **Level 1: Critical**	**Resuscitation**
Apnea or severe respiratory distress Pale, diaphoretic, and lightheaded or weak O_2 saturation <90% with oxygen Unresponsive	**Refer for immediate treatment** Many resources needed Staff at bedside Mobilization of resuscitation team
●●● **Level 2: High Risk**	**Emergent**

Altered mental status
Chest, neck, arm, or jaw pain
Difficulty breathing
Facial cyanosis or pallor
Possible overdose of beta blockers, thyroid
   medications, digoxin, or tricyclic
   antidepressants
Systolic BP <90
Dizziness or lightheadedness
Unsteady ambulation
Diaphoresis
	Do not delay treatment
	Notify physician
	Multiple diagnostic studies or procedures
	Frequent consultation
	Constant monitoring

●●● **Level 3: Moderate Risk**	**Urgent**

New medication
Unexplained weight gain, fatigue, chronically
   feeling "cold"
History of heart disease, heart block, or
   pacemaker malfunction
Nausea/vomiting
Irregular HR
	Refer for treatment as soon as possible
	May need multiple diagnostic studies or
	   procedures
	Monitor for change in condition
	If vital signs abnormal, consider Level 2

Acuity Level/Assessment	Nursing Considerations
Level 4: Low Risk	**Semi-Urgent**
HR usually slow Athletic conditioning	Reassess while waiting, per facility protocol Offer comfort measures May need a simple diagnostic study or procedure
Level 5: Lower Risk	Non-Urgent
Asymptomatic but parent or patient concerned	Reassess while waiting, per facility protocol Offer comfort measures May need examination only

RELATED PROTOCOLS:

Breathing Problems • Chest Pain • Lightheadedness/Fainting

Notes

Heat Exposure

? KEY QUESTIONS:
Name • Age • Onset • Temperature • Cardiac History • Hypertension • Diabetes • Vital Signs • Oxygen Saturation • Medications • Prior History

Acuity Level/Assessment	Nursing Considerations
Level 1: Critical	**Resuscitation**
Apnea or severe respiratory distress Pulseless Unresponsive	**Refer for immediate treatment** Staff at bedside Mobilization of resuscitation team Many resources needed
Level 2: High Risk	**Emergent**
Confusion, lethargy, disorientation Altered mental status Profuse sweating with rapid heart rate (heat exhaustion) Signs of cardiovascular collapse/shock (low BP, increased HR, increased RR) Skin hot and dry with no sweating (heatstroke) Seizures	**Do not delay treatment** Notify physician Multiple diagnostic studies or procedures Frequent consultation Continuous monitoring
Level 3: Moderate Risk	**Urgent**
Severe pain Muscle cramps or loss of coordination Vomiting Dark yellow or orange urine Dizziness, faintness, weakness Age <10 yr or >70 yr	**Refer for treatment as soon as possible** Monitor for changes in condition May need multiple diagnostic studies or procedures If alert, encourage cold liquid intake Do not give acetaminophen or aspirin to lower temperature Place patient in cool, shady area If abnormal vital signs, consider Level 2

Acuity Level/Assessment	Nursing Considerations
Level 4: Low Risk	**Semi-Urgent**
Headache Nausea Flushing	Reassess while waiting, per facility protocol Offer comfort measures May need simple diagnostic study or procedure
Level 5: Lower Risk	Non-Urgent
Symptoms improved with intake of oral fluids Asymptomatic	Reassess while waiting, per facility protocol Offer comfort measures May need an examination only

Notes

Hip Pain and Swelling

Acuity Level/Assessment	Nursing Considerations
Level 1: Critical	**Resuscitation**
Unresponsive Pulseless Apnea or severe respiratory distress	**Refer for immediate treatment** Many resources needed Staff at bedside Mobilization of resuscitation team
Level 2: High Risk	**Emergent**
Altered mental status Blue or gray foot/toes on affected side External or internal rotation and decreased motion, sensation, or circulation distally	**Do not delay treatment** Notify physician Multiple diagnostic studies or procedures Frequent consultation Constant monitoring
Level 3: Moderate Risk	**Urgent**
History of injury or fall External rotation of foot Immobility or deformity Severe pain Shortened limb Injury and history of bleeding problems Ecchymosis	**Refer for treatment as soon as possible** May need multiple diagnostic studies or procedures Monitor for change in condition If vital signs abnormal, consider Level 2
Level 4: Low Risk	**Semi-Urgent**
Moderate pain with movement	Reassess while waiting, per facility protocol Offer comfort measures May need a simple diagnostic study or procedure

Acuity Level/Assessment	Nursing Considerations
Level 5: Lower Risk	Non-Urgent
Chronic hip or joint pain Pain increases with activity Pain relieved by OTC medications	Reassess while waiting, per facility protocol Offer comfort measures May need examination only

RELATED PROTOCOLS:
Extremity Injury

Notes

Hives

KEY QUESTIONS:

Name • Age • Onset • Allergies • Prior History • Severity of Symptoms • Pain Scale • Suspected Cause • Medications • Vital Signs • Recent Changes in Food or Medication

Acuity Level/Assessment	Nursing Considerations
Level 1: Critical	**Resuscitation**
Severe difficulty breathing Unresponsive Pale, diaphoretic and lightheaded, or weak Unable to speak Severe swelling of tongue or throat	**Immediate treatment** Staff at bedside Mobilization of resuscitation team Many resources needed
Level 2: High Risk	**Emergent**
Altered mental status Prior anaphalaxis requiring epinephrine Urticaria and hives throughout body Speaking in short words Hives and rapidly progressing: Drooling Difficulty swallowing Difficulty breathing Wheezing Chest tightness Swelling of tongue or throat	**Do not delay treatment** Notify physician Multiple diagnostic studies or procedures Frequent consultation Continuous monitoring
Level 3: Moderate Risk	**Urgent**
Nausea or vomiting Abdominal pain/diarrhea Severe pain or distress Lightheadedness Facial or lip swelling Inability to speak in full sentences Contact with known allergen	**Refer for treatment as soon as possible** Monitor for change in condition May need a breathing treatment while waiting, per facility protocol May need multiple diagnostic studies or procedures If vital signs abnormal, consider Level 2

Acuity Level/Assessment	Nursing Considerations
Level 4: Low Risk	**Semi-Urgent**
Swelling of extremities Diarrhea Speaking in full sentences Hives respond to antihistamines New onset with emotional stimulus Moderate discomfort	Reassess while waiting, per facility protocol Offer comfort measures May need a simple diagnostic study or procedure
Level 5: Lower Risk	Non-Urgent
History of a viral illness Hives have resolved	Reassess while waiting, per facility protocol Offer comfort measures May need an examination only

RELATED PROTOCOLS:

Allergic Reaction • Bee Sting • Breathing Problems • Rash, Adult and Pediatric

Notes

Hypertension

Acuity Level/Assessment	Nursing Considerations
Level 1: Critical	**Resuscitation**
Apnea or severe respiratory distress Unresponsive Pulseless Pale, diaphoretic, and lightheaded or weak	**Refer for immediate treatment** Staff at bedside Mobilization of resuscitation team Many resources needed
Level 2: High Risk	**Emergent**
Altered mental status Severe weakness History of thoracic or abdominal dissection Persistent numbness and tingling in hands and feet Coughing up blood or blood-tinged sputum Difficulty breathing Persistent nosebleed Diastolic blood pressure >140 mm Hg Severe headache, blurred vision, nausea, or vomiting Chest, neck, shoulders, jaw, or back pain	**Refer for treatment within minutes** Notify physician Administer O_2 per facility protocol Perform EKG per facility protocol Administer IV per facility protocol Many diagnostic studies or procedures Frequent consultation Continuous monitoring
Level 3: Moderate Risk	**Urgent**
History of heart disease, diabetes, congestive heart failure, or blood-clotting problems	**Refer for treatment as soon as possible** Monitor for changes in condition May need multiple diagnostic studies or procedures If abnormal vital signs, consider Level 2 Consider EKG per facility protocol

Acuity Level/Assessment	Nursing Considerations
Level 4: Low Risk	**Semi-Urgent**
Periods of dizziness after starting new blood pressure medication Receiving treatment for hypertension and persistent blood pressure >160/100 mm Hg Intermittent nosebleed Strong family history of heart disease, heart attack, stroke, or diabetes	Reassess while waiting, per facility protocol Offer comfort measures May need simple diagnostic study or procedure
Level 5: Lower Risk	Non-Urgent
Persistent blood pressure readings >140/90 mm Hg	Reassess while waiting, per facility protocol Offer comfort measures May need examination only

RELATED PROTOCOLS:
Breathing Problems • Chest Pain

Notes

Itching Without a Rash

KEY QUESTIONS:

Name • Age • Onset • Allergies • Medications • Prior History • Severity of Symptoms • Pain Scale • Vital Signs

Acuity Level/Assessment	Nursing Considerations
●●● **Level 1: Critical**	**Resuscitation**
Severe respiratory distress Hypotension Unresponsive	**Refer for immediate treatment** Many resources needed Staff at bedside Mobilization of resuscitation team
●●● **Level 2: High Risk**	**Emergent**
Altered mental status	**Do not delay treatment** Notify physician Multiple diagnostic studies or procedures Frequent consultation Constant monitoring
●●● **Level 3: Moderate Risk**	**Urgent**

Itching started after taking new medication
Severe pain
Onset occurred after exposure to a known
    allergen
Recent drug withdrawal
	Refer for treatment as soon as possible
	May need multiple diagnostic studies or
	    procedures
	Monitor for change in condition
	If vital signs abnormal, consider Level 2

●●● Level 4: Low Risk	Semi-Urgent
Jaundiced skin Persistent itching Open wounds from scratching Vaginal itching	Reassess while waiting, per facility protocol Offer comfort measures May need a simple diagnostic study or procedure

Acuity Level/Assessment	Nursing Considerations
Level 5: Lower Risk	Non-Urgent
Generalized itching Itching around genitals Lice, crabs, or nits present Contact dermatitis Exposure to poison ivy or oak Rectal itching	Reassess while waiting, per facility protocol Offer comfort measures May need examination only

RELATED PROTOCOLS:
Rectal Problems

Notes

Jaundice

Acuity Level/Assessment	Nursing Considerations
● ● ● Level 1: Critical	**Resuscitation**
Severe difficulty breathing Pale, diaphoretic, and lightheaded or weak Unresponsive	**Immediate treatment** Many resources needed Staff at bedside Mobilization of resuscitation team
● ● ● Level 2: High Risk	**Emergent**
Altered mental status	**Do not delay treatment** Notify physician Multiple diagnostic studies or procedures Frequent consultation Continuous monitoring
● ● ● Level 3: Moderate Risk	**Urgent**
Malnutrition and weight loss Signs of dehydration Fever Immunosuppressed, diabetic, or pregnant Severe pain	**Refer for treatment as soon as possible** Monitor for changes in condition May need multiple diagnostic studies or procedures If abnormal vital signs, consider Level 2
● ● ● Level 4: Low Risk	**Semi-Urgent**

Known or suspected exposure to blood
  borne pathogens
Dark urine
Clay-colored stools
Vomiting
Abdominal pain
Loss of appetite
Age <10 yr or >70 yr
New onset but no other symptoms
	Reassess while waiting, per facility protocol
	Offer comfort measures
	May need a simple diagnostic study or
	  procedure

Acuity Level/Assessment	Nursing Considerations
Level 5: Lower Risk	Non-Urgent
Prior history of jaundice and no other symptoms	Reassess while waiting, per facility protocol Offer comfort measures May need an examination only

RELATED PROTOCOLS:
Abdominal Pain, Adult • Fever • Itching Without a Rash

Notes

Jaundice, Newborn

Acuity Level/Assessment	Nursing Considerations
Level 1: Critical	**Resuscitation**
Apnea or severe respiratory distress Unresponsive Pale and weak or not moving	**Immediate treatment** Many resources needed Staff at bedside Mobilization of resuscitation team
Level 2: High Risk	**Emergent**
Altered mental status Jaundice below the waistline	**Do not delay treatment** Notify physician Multiple diagnostic studies or procedures Frequent consultation Continuous monitoring
Level 3: Moderate Risk	**Urgent**
No wet diapers >8 hr Decreased oral intake Decreased activity Signs of dehydration: poor skin turgor, sunken eyes or fontanel, crying without tears Fever >100.4°F (38.0°C) Temperature <96.8°F (36.0°C)	**Refer for treatment as soon as possible** Monitor for changes in condition May need multiple diagnostic studies or procedures If abnormal vital signs, consider Level 2
Level 4: Low Risk	**Semi-Urgent**
Worsening jaundice >7 days No stool >24 hr Stools white, yellow, or gray	Reassess while waiting, per facility protocol Offer comfort measures May need a simple diagnostic study or procedure

Acuity Level/Assessment	Nursing Considerations
••• Level 5: Lower Risk	Non-Urgent
No other symptoms but parents concerned Onset of jaundice after 7 days of age	Reassess while waiting, per facility protocol Offer comfort measures May need an examination only

RELATED PROTOCOLS:
Abdominal Pain, Pediatric • Fever • Rash

Notes

Knee Pain and Swelling

Acuity Level/Assessment	Nursing Considerations
●●● Level 1: Critical	**Resuscitation**
Apnea or severe respiratory distress Unresponsive Pale, diaphoretic, and lightheaded or weak Pulseless	**Refer for immediate treatment** Staff at bedside Mobilization of resuscitation team Many resources needed
●●● Level 2: High Risk	**Emergent**
Altered mental status Cyanosis of foot or leg on affected side Chest pain Difficulty breathing Pale, paralyzed, or markedly weak leg	**Do not delay treatment** Notify physician Multiple diagnostic studies or procedures Frequent consultation Continuous monitoring
●●● Level 3: Moderate Risk	**Urgent**
Severe pain History of acute trauma Obvious deformity Leg numb	**Refer for treatment as soon as possible** May need multiple diagnostic studies or procedures Monitor for change in condition Offer wheelchair and elevate extremity Offer ice pack for known injury If vital signs abnormal, consider Level 2
●●● Level 4: Low Risk	**Semi-Urgent**
Moderate pain Inability to bear weight Red, swollen, hot joint Pain and swelling increasing with activity	Offer comfort measures Reassess while waiting, per facility protocol May need simple diagnostic study or procedure

Acuity Level/Assessment	Nursing Considerations
Level 5: Lower Risk	Non-Urgent
Chronic or intermittent pain or swelling Knee buckling or locking	Offer comfort measures Reassess while waiting, per facility protocol May need examination only

RELATED PROTOCOLS:
Extremity Injury

Notes

Laceration

KEY QUESTIONS:

Name • Age • Onset • Allergies • Medications • Prior History • Mechanism of Injury • Severity • Pain Scale • Vital Signs • Last Tetanus Immunization

Acuity Level/Assessment	Nursing Considerations
●●● **Level 1: Critical**	**Resuscitation**
Apnea or severe respiratory distress Pulseless Unresponsive Pale, diaphoretic, and lightheaded or weak	**Refer for immediate treatment** Staff at bedside Mobilization of resuscitation team Many resources needed
●●● **Level 2: High Risk**	**Emergent**
Altered mental status Pulsatile bleeding Exposure of deep structures (tissue, tendons, organs, bone, etc.) Laceration near a major artery No pulse distal to laceration Cyanotic distal to laceration Impaled object Gaping, bleeding wound	**Do not delay treatment** Notify physician Multiple diagnostic studies or procedures Frequent consultation Continuous monitoring Apply compression dressing to control bleeding Leave impaled object in place
●●● **Level 3: Moderate Risk**	**Urgent**
Severe pain Gaping wound with bleeding controlled History of bleeding disorder Laceration involves a joint Decreased range of motion of the limb Facial laceration	**Refer for treatment as soon as possible** Reassess, per facility protocol May need multiple diagnostic studies or procedures Monitor for changes in condition If vital signs abnormal, consider Level 2
●●● **Level 4: Low Risk**	**Semi-Urgent**
Moderate pain Taking anticoagulant Signs of infection	Reassess while waiting, per facility protocol Offer comfort measures May need simple diagnostic study or procedure

Acuity Level/Assessment	Nursing Considerations
●●● **Level 4: Low Risk**	**Semi-Urgent**
Road abrasions Stable laceration(s) with bleeding controlled, awaiting cleaning and suturing	
●●● Level 5: Lower Risk	Non-Urgent
Minor laceration in need of cleaning and minimal repair	Reassess while waiting, per facility protocol Offer comfort measures May need examination only

RELATED PROTOCOLS:
Wound Infection

Notes

Lightheadedness/Fainting

Acuity Level/Assessment	Nursing Considerations
● ● ● Level 1: Critical	**Resuscitation**
Apnea or severe respiratory distress Pulseless Unresponsive Pale, diaphoretic, and lightheaded or weak	**Immediate treatment** Staff at bedside Mobilization of resuscitation team Many resources needed
● ● ● Level 2: High Risk	**Emergent**
Severe pain Confusion, lethargy, disorientation Altered mental status Weakness or inability to move arms or legs Difficulty speaking, disturbed vision Irregular HR or palpitations Chest pain	**Do not delay treatment** Notify physician Multiple diagnostic studies or procedures Frequent consultation Continuous monitoring
● ● ● Level 3: Moderate Risk	**Urgent**
Recent head trauma with nausea or vomiting Moderate to severe vomiting or diarrhea Bleeding and tachycardia Postural vital signs Persistent headache or change in vision Diabetes	**Refer for treatment as soon as possible** Monitor for changes in condition May need multiple diagnostic studies or procedures Measure serum glucose level If abnormal vital signs, consider Level 2
● ● ● Level 4: Low Risk	**Semi-Urgent**
Symptoms interfere with activities Symptoms occur after taking new medication Symptoms occur with head movement Pregnancy or LMP >6 wk previous Exposure to sun or hot environment Earache, tinnitus, loss of hearing	Reassess while waiting, per facility protocol Offer comfort measures May need a simple diagnostic study or procedure

Acuity Level/Assessment	Nursing Considerations
Level 5: Lower Risk	Non-Urgent
History of dieting Increased stress, emotional event, or hyperventilation Symptoms occur with alcohol consumption	Reassess while waiting, per facility protocol Offer comfort measures May need an examination only

RELATED PROTOCOLS:

Altered Mental Status • Abdominal Pain, Adult • Abdominal Pain, Pediatric • Chest Pain • Diarrhea, Adult • Diarrhea, Pediatric • Headache • Vaginal Bleeding, Abnormal • Vomiting

Notes

Menstrual Problems

KEY QUESTIONS:
Name • Age • Onset • Allergies • Medications • Prior History • Severity • Pain Scale • Vital Signs • Number of Saturated Pads or Tampons Per Hour • Birth Control • Possibility of Pregnancy

Acuity Level/Assessment	Nursing Considerations
Level 1: Critical	**Resuscitation**
Apnea or severe respiratory distress Unresponsive Pale, diaphoretic, and lightheaded or weak Pulseless	**Refer for immediate treatment** Staff at bedside Mobilization of resuscitation team Many resources needed
Level 2: High Risk	**Emergent**
Altered mental status Hypotensive Partial or complete expulsion of products of conception Persistent bleeding saturating >2 regular-size pads or tampons per hour >2 hr Severe pain and possibility of pregnancy Sexually active and last period >6 wk prior and abdominal or shoulder pain	**Do not delay treatment** Notify physician Multiple diagnostic studies or procedures Frequent consultation Continuous monitoring
Level 3: Moderate Risk	**Urgent**
Severe pain Heavy vaginal bleeding with clots Saturating 1 regular-size pad per hour >6 hr Fainting or lightheadedness sitting or standing up Use of tampons and sudden high fever, sunburn-type rash, general ill feeling, lightheadedness, vomiting, watery diarrhea, tachycardia, or headache	**Refer for treatment as soon as possible** May need multiple diagnostic studies or procedures Monitor for changes in condition If vital signs abnormal, consider Level 2

Acuity Level/Assessment	Nursing Considerations
Level 4: Low Risk	**Semi-Urgent**
Cramping interferes with daily activity Persistent vaginal discharge Persistent vaginal bleeding >10 days or <21 days since last period Possible pregnancy, bleeding, and no pain No menses and taking birth control pills	Offer comfort measures Reassess while waiting, per facility protocol May need simple diagnostic study or procedure
Level 5: Lower Risk	Non-Urgent
Unusually heavy menstrual flow Scant menstruation Period missed or delayed and age >40 y	Offer comfort measures Reassess while waiting, per facility protocol May need examination only

RELATED PROTOCOLS:
Abdominal Pain, Adult • Vaginal Bleeding, Abnormal

Notes

Motor Vehicle Accident

KEY QUESTIONS:
Name • Age • Onset • Allergies • Prior History • Severity • Pain Scale • Vital Signs • Oxygen Saturation • Extent of Injuries

Acuity Level/Assessment	Nursing Considerations
●●● **Level 1: Critical**	**Resuscitation**
Apnea or severe respiratory distress Pulseless Unresponsive High risk: mechanism of injury Pale, diaphoretic, and lightheaded or weak	**Refer for immediate treatment** Staff at bedside Mobilization of resuscitation team C-spine immobilization Many resources needed
●●● **Level 2: High Risk**	**Emergent**
Altered mental status Uncontrolled bleeding High rate of speed Unrestrained in vehicle Bruising over vital organs Multiple large lacerations Point tenderness High risk medical history (diabetes, cancer, hemophilia, etc.)	**Do not delay treatment** Notify physician Multiple diagnostic studies or procedures Frequent consultation Continuous monitoring C-spine immobilization
●●● **Level 3: Moderate Risk**	**Urgent**
Severe pain Ambulatory at scene of a minor MVA Small lacerations with bleeding controlled Moderate risk Mechanism of injury	**Refer for treatment as soon as possible** May need multiple diagnostic studies or procedures Monitor for changes in condition If vital signs abnormal, consider Level 2

Acuity Level/Assessment	Nursing Considerations
Level 4: Low Risk	**Semi-Urgent**
Moderate pain Minor bruising or aches Minor lacerations or abrasions with bleeding controlled	Offer comfort measures Reassess while waiting, per facility protocol May need simple diagnostic study or procedure If other occupant of same vehicle was a fatality, consider Level 3
Level 5: Lower Risk	Non-Urgent
No complaints of pain, bruising, or injury from a low-speed, minor MVA >24 hr since MVA (with no major complaints)	Offer comfort measures Reassess while waiting, per facility protocol May need examination only

RELATED PROTOCOLS:

Ankle Pain and Swelling • Back Pain • Cold Exposure, Hypothermia/Frostbite • Extremity Injury • Head Injury • Knee Pain and Swelling • Neck Pain • Puncture Wound • Shoulder Pain

See Appendix J: MVA Triage Questions; Appendix K: Mechanisms of Injury from Trauma: Adult; Appendix L: Mechanisms of Injury: School Age and Adolescent; Appendix M: Mechanisms of Injury: Toddler and Preschooler; Appendix N: Mechanisms of Injury: Infant

Notes

Mouth Problems

Acuity Level/Assessment	Nursing Considerations
●●● **Level 1: Critical**	**Resuscitation**
Apnea or severe respiratory distress Pulseless Unresponsive Sudden swelling in back of throat or tongue Injury impedes airway Pale, diaphoretic, and lightheaded or weak	**Refer for immediate treatment** Staff at bedside Mobilization of resuscitation team Many resources needed
●●● **Level 2: High Risk**	**Emergent**
Altered mental status Inability to open/close mouth, jaw locked in place Penetrating injury to the back of the mouth Uncontrolled bleeding Traumatic injury that may potentially impede airway "Kissing tonsils" (unable to swallow own saliva) Drooling Tongue amputation	**Do not delay treatment** Notify physician Multiple diagnostic studies or procedures Frequent consultation Continuous monitoring Maintain airway
●●● **Level 3: Moderate Risk**	**Urgent**
Severe pain not relieved with OTC medications or ice pack Gaping lacerations Facial swelling with unobstructed airway "Kissing tonsils" (able to swallow own saliva) Difficulty speaking Pain with facial swelling	**Refer for treatment as soon as possible** May need multiple diagnostic studies or procedures Monitor for change in condition Control bleeding If vital signs abnormal, consider Level 2

Acuity Level/Assessment	Nursing Considerations
Level 4: Low Risk	**Semi-Urgent**
Moderate pain Foul taste is or odor from mouth Open sores, blisters, or white patches Fever and mouth sores	Offer comfort measures Reassess while waiting, per facility protocol May need simple diagnostic study or procedure
Level 5: Lower Risk	Non-Urgent
Dental caries and pain Red or tender gums Sore spot on tongue	Offer comfort measures Reassess while waiting, per facility protocol May need examination only

RELATED PROTOCOLS:

Breathing Problems • Sore Throat • Toothache/Tooth Injury

Notes

Neck Pain

Name • Age • Onset • Allergies • Medications • Prior History • Mechanism of Injury • Pain Scale • Vital Signs • Oxygen Saturation

Acuity Level/Assessment	Nursing Considerations
●●● Level 1: Critical	**Resuscitation**
Apnea or severe respiratory distress Pulseless Unresponsive High risk mechanism of injury with neurological deficits Pale, diaphoretic, and lightheaded or weak	**Refer for immediate treatment** Staff at bedside Mobilization of resuscitation team Many resources needed
●●● Level 2: High Risk	**Emergent**
Altered mental status High risk mechanism of injury with no neurological deficits Sudden onset of chest, jaw, or neck pain (no known injury) Difficulty breathing Severe headache and fever >101.3°F (38.5°C) Petechiae Sudden onset of numbness, tingling, weakness in both arms or legs Diaphoresis, palpitations, nausea, and/or vomiting Severe pain	**Do not delay treatment** Notify physician Multiple diagnostic studies or procedures Frequent consultation Continuous monitoring
●●● Level 3: Moderate Risk	**Urgent**
Neck pain worsens with flexion Low risk mechanism of injury Photophobia Nausea and vomiting Weakness or numbness in one arm	**Refer for treatment as soon as possible** May need multiple diagnostic studies or procedures Monitor for changes in condition If vital signs abnormal, consider Level 2

Acuity Level/Assessment	Nursing Considerations
Level 4: Low Risk	Semi-Urgent
Moderate neck pain worsens with extension Swollen glands, sore throat, cold symptoms, earache Swelling on one or both sides of neck Pain interferes with daily activity	Offer comfort measures Reassess while waiting, per facility protocol May need simple diagnostic study or procedure
Level 5: Lower Risk	Non-Urgent
Neck pain without history of trauma or illness Chronic neck pain Slept in awkward position	Offer comfort measures Reassess while waiting, per facility protocol May need examination only

RELATED PROTOCOLS:

Chest Pain • Ear Problems • Fever • Head Injury • Sore Throat • Toothache/Tooth Injury

Notes

Nosebleed

KEY QUESTIONS:
Name • Age • Onset • Allergies • Prior History • Medications • Pain Scale • Vital Signs • Oxygen Saturation

Acuity Level/Assessment	Nursing Considerations
●●● **Level 1: Critical**	**Resuscitation**
Apnea or severe respiratory distress Pulseless Unresponsive Pale, diaphoretic, dizzy, or weak	**Refer for immediate treatment** Staff at bedside Mobilization of resuscitation team Many resources needed
●●● **Level 2: High Risk**	**Emergent**
Altered mental status Abnormal vital signs Uncontrolled bleeding with clots	**Do not delay treatment** Notify physician Multiple diagnostic studies or procedures Frequent consultation Continuous monitoring Provide IV access per facility protocol Lab draw, consider blood type and cross per facility protocol
●●● **Level 3: Moderate Risk**	**Urgent**
Severe pain Moderate to heavy bleeding (anterior bleed) Bleeding from nasal or facial trauma Hemoptysis Bleeding uncontrolled after 30 min of direct pressure History of bleeding disorder or other hematologic disease (leukemia, thrombocytopenia, etc.) and intermittant nosebleeds Headache Normal vital signs and lightheadedness	**Refer for treatment as soon as possible** May need multiple diagnostic studies or procedures Monitor for change in condition If abnormal vital signs, consider Level 2 Instruct patient to gently blow through the nose to clear nares Administer nasal spray to help control bleeding, per facility protocol Clamp nose for 10 min

Acuity Level/Assessment	Nursing Considerations
●●● **Level 4: Low Risk**	**Semi-Urgent**
Intermittent nosebleed (>3 in past 48 hours) Recent nasal surgery Frequent use of cocaine Moderate pain	Reassess while waiting, per facility protocol Offer comfort measures May need a simple diagnostic study or procedure
●●● Level 5: Lower Risk	Non-Urgent
Seasonal allergies Frequent use of nasal sprays History of frequent controlled nosebleeds	Reassess while waiting, per facility protocol Offer comfort measures May need an examination only

RELATED PROTOCOLS:
Cold Symptoms • Foreign Body, Inhaled

Notes

Poisoning, Exposure or Ingestion

KEY QUESTIONS:
Name • Age • Weight • Onset • Amount • Emesis After Ingestion • Allergies • Prior History • Medications • Pain Scale • Vital Signs • Oxygen Saturation • Name of Agent (if Known)

Acuity Level/Assessment	Nursing Considerations
Level 1: Critical	**Resuscitation**
Apnea or severe respiratory distress Pulseless Unresponsive Status epilepticus	**Refer for immediate treatment** Staff at bedside Mobilization of resuscitation team Many resources needed Contact National Poison Control Center for advice (1-800-222-1222)
Level 2: High Risk	**Emergent**
Altered mental status Lethargy Chest pain Recent seizure or postictal Wheezing, stridor, shortness of breath Ingestion of an acid, alkali, or hydrocarbon agent Burns on lips or tongue Cyanosis Unstable vital signs Suicide attempt Constricted or dilated pupils Known carbon monoxide exposure Strong suspicion of exposure to WMD agent and symptomatic Excessive drooling or sweating or hyperactive reflexes Fever >104°F (40.0°C) Child found with open medication bottle or other potentially dangerous substances	**Do not delay treatment** Notify physician Multiple diagnostic studies or procedures Frequent consultation Continuous monitoring Contact National Poison Control Center for advice (1-800-222-1222) Provide IV access, perform EKG, per facility protocol If suicide attempt, place in observed area until bed available If multiple patients with similar symptoms, consider WMD exposure and initiate decontamination procedures per facility plan

Acuity Level/Assessment	Nursing Considerations
●●● **Level 3: Moderate Risk**	**Urgent**

Severe pain
Nausea, vomiting, diarrhea
Abdominal pain
Headache
Ataxia
Dizziness or lightheadedness
Psychiatric history
Cognitive dysfunction
Irritability
Smell of chemical on breath or clothes
	Refer for treatment as soon as possible
	May need multiple diagnostic studies or
	  procedures
	Monitor for changes in condition
	If vital signs abnormal, consider Level 2
	Contact National Poison Control Center for
	  advice (1-800-222-1222)

●●● **Level 4: Low Risk**	**Semi-Urgent**

Moderate pain
Poison oak or poison ivy exposure and
  urticaria and rash
	Reassess while waiting, per facility protocol
	Offer comfort measures
	May need simple diagnostic study or procedure
	Contact National Poison Control Center for
	  advice (1-800-222-1222)

●●● Level 5: Lower Risk	Non-Urgent

Gave twice the recommended amount of OTC
  medication
Asymptomatic but parent or patient concerned
	Reassess while waiting, per facility protocol
	Offer comfort measures
	May need examination only
	Contact National Poison Control Center for
	  advice (1-800-222-1222)

RELATED PROTOCOLS:

Alcohol and Drug Use, Abuse, and Dependence • Bites, Insect and Tick • Bites, Marine Animal • Bites, Snake • Suicidal Behavior

See Appendix Q, Biological Agents/Chemical Agents; Appendix O, Drugs of Abuse; Appendix P: Poisonings

Pregnancy, Abdominal Pain

KEY QUESTIONS:
Name • Age • Onset • Allergies • Prior History • Severity • Pain Scale • Vital Signs • Oxygen Saturation • Gestational Age • Recent Ultrasound • Number of Pregnancies

Acuity Level/Assessment	Nursing Considerations
●●● **Level 1: Critical**	**Resuscitation**
Apnea or severe respiratory distress Imminent delivery, crowning noted Seizure Ruptured membranes with prolapsed cord Pale, diaphoretic, and lightheaded or weak	**Refer for immediate treatment** Staff at bedside Mobilization of resuscitation team Many resources needed Monitor fetal heart tones
●●● **Level 2: High Risk**	**Emergent**
Altered mental status No fetal movement with gestational age >24 wk Passing tissue with heavy vaginal bleeding Painful vaginal bleeding (abruptio placentae) and pregnancy >20 wk Contractions every 2 to 3 min (precipitous birth) and pregnancy >20 wk	**Do not delay treatment** Notify physician Multiple diagnostic studies or procedures Frequent consultation Continuous monitoring If pregnancy >20 wk, transfer to labor and delivery, per facility protocol Monitor fetal heart tones
●●● **Level 3: Moderate Risk**	**Urgent**
Painless vaginal bleeding (placenta previa) and pregnancy >20 wk First trimester of pregnancy (ectopic) Twenty to 37 wk gestation (preterm labor) Nausea, vomiting, diarrhea Bright red emesis, stools, or hematuria Sudden weight gain, edema, headache History of prior pregnancy complications Fever >102.2°F (>39.0°C)	**Refer for treatment as soon as possible** May need multiple diagnostic studies or procedures Monitor for changes in condition If vital signs abnormal, consider Level 2 Postural vital signs If pregnancy >20 wk, transfer to labor and delivery, per facility protocol Monitor fetal heart tones

Acuity Level/Assessment	Nursing Considerations
Level 4: Low Risk	**Semi-Urgent**
Moderate pain Frequent urination or burning Fever, cough, earache, sore throat Vaginal discharge	Offer comfort measures Reassess while waiting, per facility protocol May need simple diagnostic study or procedure
Level 5: Lower Risk	Non-Urgent
Heartburn "Morning sickness"	Offer comfort measures Reassess while waiting, per facility protocol May need examination only

RELATED PROTOCOLS:

Pregnancy, Back Pain • Pregnancy, Vaginal Bleeding • Pregnancy, Vaginal Discharge

Notes

Pregnancy, Back Pain

KEY QUESTIONS:
Name • Age • Onset • Allergies • Prior History • Severity • Pain Scale • Vital Signs • Oxygen Saturation • Gestational Age • Recent Ultrasound • Number of Pregnancies

Acuity Level/Assessment	Nursing Considerations
●●● **Level 1: Critical**	**Resuscitation**
Apnea or severe respiratory distress Unresponsive Imminent delivery, crowning noted Seizure Ruptured membranes with prolapsed cord Pale, diaphoretic, and lightheaded or weak	**Refer for immediate treatment** Staff at bedside Mobilization of resuscitation team Many resources needed Monitor fetal heart tones Place in knee-chest or Trendelenburg position Check cord for pulsation
●●● **Level 2: High Risk**	**Emergent**
Altered mental status Contractions and <37 wk gestation No fetal movement Strong, regular contractions Recent trauma	**Do not delay treatment** Notify physician Multiple diagnostic studies or procedures Frequent consultation Continuous monitoring If pregnancy >20 wk, transfer to labor and delivery, per facility protocol Monitor fetal heart tones
●●● **Level 3: Moderate Risk**	**Urgent**

Fever >102.2°F (>39.0°C)
Urinary frequency, burning, hematuria
Difficulty starting a urine stream
Flank pain
Rectal pain
Right upper quadrant pain or shoulder pain
Multigravida and history of prior pregnancy
    complications
	Refer for treatment as soon as possible
	May need multiple diagnostic studies or
	    procedures
	Monitor for changes in condition
	If vital signs abnormal, consider Level 2
	Orthostatic vital signs
	If pregnancy >20 wk, transfer to labor and
	    delivery, per facility protocol
	Monitor fetal heart tones

Acuity Level/Assessment	Nursing Considerations
Level 4: Low Risk	**Semi-Urgent**
Moderate pain Musculoskeletal pain	Offer comfort measures Reassess while waiting, per facility protocol May need simple diagnostic study or procedure
Level 5: Lower Risk	Non-Urgent
Mild pain associated with increase in activity	Offer comfort measures Reassess while waiting, per facility protocol May need examination only

RELATED PROTOCOLS:

Pregnancy, Abdominal Pain • Pregnancy, Vaginal Bleeding • Pregnancy, Vaginal Discharge

Notes

Pregnancy, Vaginal Bleeding

Name • Age • Onset • Allergies • Prior History • Severity • Pain Scale • Vital Signs • Last Menstrual Period • Number of Regular-Size Saturated Pads • Medications

Acuity Level/Assessment	Nursing Considerations
●●● Level 1: Critical	**Resuscitation**
Apnea or severe respiratory distress Pulseless Unresponsive Prolapsed cord Pale, diaphoretic, and lightheaded	**Refer for immediate treatment** Staff at bedside Mobilization of resuscitation team Many resources needed Monitor fetal heart tones Place in knee-chest or Trendelenburg position Check cord for pulsation
●●● Level 2: High Risk	**Emergent**
Altered mental status Profuse, bright red blood and pregnancy >20 wk Passing large clots or products of conception Painful vaginal bleeding (abruptio placentae) Hypotension or tachycardia Severe abdominal pain Lightheadedness No fetal movement and pregnancy >20 wk Known trauma	**Do not delay treatment** Notify physician Multiple diagnostic studies or procedures Frequent consultation Continuous monitoring If pregnancy >20 wk, transfer to labor and delivery, per facility protocol Monitor fetal heart tones Position patient on left side
●●● Level 3: Moderate Risk	**Urgent**
Severe pain Painless vaginal bleeding and pregnancy >20 wk Moderate flow, bright red blood (placenta previa) Strong, regular contractions Leaking clear fluid <10 fetal movements in 1 hr	**Refer for treatment as soon as possible** May need multiple diagnostic studies or procedures Monitor for changes in condition If vital signs abnormal, consider Level 2 Postural vital signs If pregnancy >20 wk, transfer to labor and delivery, per facility protocol Monitor fetal heart tones

Acuity Level/Assessment	Nursing Considerations
Level 4: Low Risk	**Semi-Urgent**
Moderate pain Minimal bleeding but patient concerned	Offer comfort measures Reassess while waiting, per facility protocol May need simple diagnostic study or procedure
Level 5: Lower Risk	Non-Urgent
Spotting dark brown or pink blood after intercourse	Offer comfort measures Reassess while waiting, per facility protocol May need examination only

RELATED PROTOCOLS:

Pregnancy, Abdominal Pain • Pregnancy, Back Pain • Pregnancy, Vaginal Discharge

Notes

Pregnancy, Vaginal Discharge

Acuity Level/Assessment	Nursing Considerations
●●● Level 1: Critical	**Resuscitation**
Apnea or severe respiratory distress Pale, diaphoretic, and lightheaded or weak Ruptured membranes with prolapsed cord	**Refer for immediate treatment** Staff at bedside Mobilization of resuscitation team Many resources needed Monitor fetal heart tones Place in knee-chest or Trendelenburg position Check cord for pulsation
●●● Level 2: High Risk	**Emergent**
Altered mental status Severe abdominal pain No fetal movement and pregnancy >20 wk Imminent delivery with crowning or meconium	**Do not delay treatment** Notify physician Multiple diagnostic studies or procedures Frequent consultation Continuous monitoring If pregnancy >20 wk, transfer to labor and delivery, per facility protocol Monitor fetal heart tones
●●● Level 3: Moderate Risk	**Urgent**
Fever >102.2°F (>39.0°C) with purulent vaginal discharge Herpes outbreak with regular contractions or leaking of fluid Green, brown, or red-stained fluid	**Refer for treatment as soon as possible** May need multiple diagnostic studies or procedures Monitor for changes in condition If vital signs abnormal, consider Level 2 Monitor fetal heart tones

Acuity Level/Assessment	Nursing Considerations
Level 4: Low Risk	**Semi-Urgent**
Moderate pain Irregular contractions History of STD exposure Clumped, white, curd-like discharge	Offer comfort measures Reassess while waiting, per facility protocol May need simple diagnostic study or procedure
Level 5: Lower Risk	Non-Urgent
Lost mucous plug Increase in vaginal mucus secretions	Offer comfort measures Reassess while waiting, per facility protocol May need examination only

RELATED PROTOCOLS:

Pregnancy, Vaginal Bleeding • Vaginal Bleeding, Abnormal

Notes

Pregnancy, Vomiting

Acuity Level/Assessment	Nursing Considerations
●●● **Level 1: Critical**	**Resuscitation**
Severe respiratory distress Pale, diaphoretic, and lightheaded Unresponsive Pale, diaphoretic, dizzy, weak	**Refer for immediate treatment** Staff at bedside Mobilization of resuscitation team Many resources needed Monitor fetal heart tones
●●● **Level 2: High Risk**	**Emergent**
Altered mental status Vomiting bright red blood Chest pain Difficulty breathing Recent head or abdominal trauma Abnormal vital signs	**Do not delay treatment** Notify physician Multiple diagnostic studies or procedures Frequent consultation Continuous monitoring Monitor fetal heart tones
●●● **Level 3: Moderate Risk**	**Urgent**
Severe pain Signs of dehydration Coffee ground emesis Diabetes and hyperglycemia or hypoglycemia Lightheadedness Orthostatic vital signs Dark, amber urine Right upper or lower quadrant pain Abdominal pain and nausea, vomiting, or diarrhea Fever >102.2°F (>39.0°C)	**Refer for treatment as soon as possible** May need multiple diagnostic studies or procedures Monitor for changes in condition Postural vital signs If vital signs abnormal, consider Level 2 Monitor fetal heart tones

Acuity Level/Assessment	Nursing Considerations
Level 4: Low Risk ● ● ●	**Semi-Urgent**
Moderate pain Nausea and vomiting associated with gastroenteritis Vomiting >24 hr (no dehydration signs)	Offer comfort measures Reassess while waiting, per facility protocol May need simple diagnostic study or procedure
Level 5: Lower Risk ● ● ●	Non-Urgent
Heartburn No other symptoms but patient concerned	Offer comfort measures Reassess while waiting, per facility protocol May need examination only

RELATED PROTOCOLS:

Pregnancy, Abdominal Pain • Vomiting

Notes

Puncture Wound

Name • Age • Onset • Allergies • Medications • Prior History • Pain Scale • Vital Signs • Tetanus Immunization Status • Mechanism of Injury (Appendices K–N)

Acuity Level/Assessment	Nursing Considerations
Level 1: Critical	**Resuscitation**
Apnea or severe respiratory distress Pulseless Unresponsive Involvement of vital organ Pale, diaphoretic, and lightheaded or weak	**Refer for immediate treatment** Staff at bedside Mobilization of resuscitation team Many resources needed
Level 2: High Risk	**Emergent**
Altered mental status High risk mechanism of injury (mass, size, and velocity of wounding object and direction of impact) Large amount of bleeding and difficult to control with pressure Pulsatile bleeding Pulses absent distal to injury Skin cyanotic distal to wound High-pressure injection injury Impaled object obvious to head or trunk	**Do not delay treatment** Notify physician Multiple diagnostic studies or procedures Frequent consultation Continuous monitoring Leave impaled object in place Apply compression dressing to control bleeding Refer to appropriate mechanism of injury resource in appendices K–N
Level 3: Moderate Risk	**Urgent**
Severe pain Paresthesia distal to injury Pulses weak distal to injury Decreased range of motion to the affected area Puncture wound in a joint Fever and chills History of bleeding disorder, cancer, etc.	**Refer for treatment as soon as possible** Reassess, per facility protocol May need multiple diagnostic studies or procedures Monitor for changes in condition If vital signs abnormal, consider Level 2 Do not soak if wood sliver

Acuity Level/Assessment	Nursing Considerations
Level 3: Moderate Risk	**Urgent**
Tip of impaled object broken off and not visible Foreign body sensation persists Impaled object obvious to an extremity	
Level 4: Low Risk	**Semi-Urgent**
Moderate pain Puncture wound through a shoe No prior tetanus prophylaxis Fever, red streaks, purulent drainage	Reassess while waiting, per facility protocol Offer comfort measures May need simple diagnostic study or procedure Do not soak if wood sliver
Level 5: Lower Risk	Non-Urgent
Small object in distal extremity No other symptoms but parent or patient concerned Tetanus prophylaxis status >5 yr	Reassess while waiting, per facility protocol Offer comfort measures May need examination only Do not soak if wood sliver

RELATED PROTOCOLS:

Bites, Animal and Human • Bites, Marine Animal • Bites, Snake • Foreign Body, Skin • Laceration • Motor Vehicle Accidents • Suicidal Behavior • Wound Infection

Notes

Rash, Adult and Pediatric

Acuity Level/Assessment	Nursing Considerations
Level 1: Critical	**Resuscitation**
Severe respiratory distress Unresponsive Pale, diaphoretic, and lightheaded or weak Anaphylaxis Pulseless	**Refer for immediate treatment** Staff at bedside Mobilization of resuscitation team Many resources needed
Level 2: High Risk	**Emergent**
Altered mental status Fever and petechiae (nonblanching) or purpura (nonblanching) Fever and severe localized pain Red skin peeling off in sheets Stiff neck, severe headache Sudden onset of hives and difficulty breathing Child with any of the following: Unusual drowsiness, refusal to drink, and noisy or fast breathing Signs of dehydration: sunken eyes or fontanel, no wet diapers Drooling	**Do not delay treatment** Notify physician Multiple diagnostic studies or procedures Frequent consultation Continuous monitoring
Level 3: Moderate Risk	**Urgent**
Severe pain Redness and swelling of the eyelid Facial swelling Fever, red rash, and using tampons or history of recent surgery Severe itching, irritation, and open skin	**Refer for treatment as soon as possible** Reassess, per facility protocol May need multiple diagnostic studies or procedures Monitor for changes in condition If vital signs abnormal, consider Level 2

Acuity Level/Assessment	Nursing Considerations
Level 4: Low Risk	**Semi-Urgent**
Moderate pain Signs of infection: redness, swelling, pain, red streaks, or drainage from wound Fever, sore throat, or cold symptoms Joint pain or swelling Exposure to poison oak or poison ivy Localized area of painful blisters Non localized fluid filled blisters Newborn with blisters Blanching petechiae or purpura and no fever Multiple lesions in mouth Rash, blisters, pimples, or crusting under diaper area	Reassess while waiting, per facility protocol Offer comfort measures May need simple diagnostic study or procedure
Level 5: Lower Risk	Non-Urgent
Dermatitis Herpes outbreak Asymptomatic rash lasting >48 hr Recent exposure to chickenpox or measles Red or weeping rash in groin or diaper area Extensive rash, cause unknown	Reassess while waiting, per facility protocol Offer comfort measures May need examination only May isolate patients with communicable disease exposure and symptomatic from other waiting patients

RELATED PROTOCOLS:

Allergic Reaction • Bites, Animal and Human • Bites, Insect and Tick • Bites, Marine Animal • Bites, Snake • Poisoning, Exposure or Ingestion

Notes

Rectal Problems (see Foreign Body, Rectum or Vagina, for foreign body problem)

(see Foreign Body, Rectum or Vagina, for foreign body problem)

KEY QUESTIONS:

Name • Age • Onset • Allergies • Medications • Prior History • Severity • Pain Scale • Vital Signs

Acuity Level/Assessment	Nursing Considerations
Level 1: Critical	**Resuscitation**
Apnea or severe respiratory distress Pale, diaphoretic, and lightheaded or weak Unresponsive Pulseless	**Refer for immediate treatment** Staff at bedside Mobilization of resuscitation team Many resources needed
Level 2: High Risk	**Emergent**
Altered mental status Heavy rectal bleeding mixed in the stool or passing of blood clots Traumatic injury to rectum by a knife or blunt object Black or bloody stools and lightheadedness Frequent black, tarry stools	**Do not delay treatment** Notify physician Multiple diagnostic studies or procedures Frequent consultation Continuous monitoring
Level 3: Moderate Risk	**Urgent**
Severe rectal pain Sexual assault Urinary retention Moderate rectal bleeding and no history of hemorrhoids; or bleeding with constipation Acute abdominal pain, bloating, nausea, or vomiting Rectal pain and fever >102.2°F (>39.0°C) Foreign body in rectum Constipation and vomiting brown, yellow, or green bitter-tasting emesis	**Refer for treatment as soon as possible** May need multiple diagnostic studies or procedures Monitor for change in condition If vital signs abnormal, consider Level 2

Acuity Level/Assessment	Nursing Considerations
Level 3: Moderate Risk	**Urgent**
Black or bloody stools and use of blood thinners, steroids, nonsteroidal anti-inflammatory medications, or large doses of aspirin	
Level 4: Low Risk	**Semi-Urgent**
Moderate rectal pain or itching that interferes with activities of daily living Minimal rectal bleeding and history of hemorrhoids or bleeding with constipation Low-grade fever or signs of infection: spreading redness, open sores, drainage Exposure to an STD Painful blisters around rectal area Last bowel movement >5 days previous Infant with no stool >6–10 days Fever, constipation and history of recent surgery, injury, childbirth, or diverticulitis	Reassess while waiting, per facility protocol Offer comfort measures May need simple diagnostic study or procedure
Level 5: Lower Risk	Non-Urgent
Worms visible in the stool Rectal itching Chronic constipation Intermittent rectal pain with bowel movements	Reassess while waiting, per facility protocol Offer comfort measures May need examination only

RELATED PROTOCOLS:

Abdominal Pain, Adult • Abdominal Pain, Pediatric • Foreign Body, Rectum/Vagina • Sexual Assault

Seizure

KEY QUESTIONS:

Name • Age • Onset • Allergies • Medications • Prior History • Severity • Pain Scale • Vital Signs • Oxygen Saturation • Drug and Alcohol Use

Acuity Level/Assessment	Nursing Considerations
● ● ● Level 1: Critical	**Resuscitation**
Apnea or severe respiratory distress Pulseless Unresponsive Status epilepticus Pale, diaphoretic, and lightheaded or weak	**Refer for immediate treatment** Staff at bedside Mobilization of resuscitation team Many resources needed
● ● ● Level 2: High Risk	**Emergent**
Altered mental status History of head injury Pregnancy: eclampsia Overdose or poisoning Sudden onset of weakness, inability to move one side of the body, difficulty speaking Strong suspicion of exposure to WMD agent and symptomatic Severe headache First-time seizure Persistent, unusual lethargy	**Do not delay treatment** Notify physician Multiple diagnostic studies or procedures Frequent consultation Continuous monitoring If multiple patients with similar symptoms or suspected exposure to WMD agent, initiate decontamination procedures, per facility plan See appendix Q, Biological Agents/Chemical Agents
● ● ● Level 3: Moderate Risk	**Urgent**
Severe pain Fever >101.4°F Sudden cessation of alcohol or drug consumption in the chronic user Frequent seizures while taking anticonvulsant medications	**Refer for treatment as soon as possible** May need multiple diagnostic studies or procedures Monitor for changes in condition If vital signs abnormal, consider Level 2

Acuity Level/Assessment	Nursing Considerations
Level 3: Moderate Risk	**Urgent**
Headache Nuchal rigidity History of seizures and inconsistent use of medications or excessive alcohol use	
Level 4: Low Risk	**Semi-Urgent**
Moderate pain History of cancer, diabetes, or immunosuppression History of seizures and out of medication	Reassess while waiting, per facility protocol Offer comfort measures May need simple diagnostic study or procedure
Level 5: Lower Risk	Non-Urgent
History of psychosomatic seizures History of seizures and alert and oriented after waking up from the seizure	Reassess while waiting, per facility protocol Offer comfort measures May need examination only

RELATED PROTOCOLS:

Altered Mental Status • Alcohol and Drug Use, Abuse, and Dependence • Bites, Animal and Human • Bites, Insect and Tick • Bites, Marine Animal • Bites, Snake • Confusion • Diabetic Problems • Fever • Head Injury • Poisoning, Exposure or Ingestion

Notes

Seizure, Pediatric Febrile

Acuity Level/Assessment	Nursing Considerations
●●● Level 1: Critical	**Resuscitation**
Apnea or severe respiratory distress Pulseless Unresponsive Status epilepticus Pale, diaphoretic, and lightheaded or weak	**Refer for immediate treatment** Staff at bedside Mobilization of resuscitation team Many resources needed
●●● Level 2: High Risk	**Emergent**
Altered mental status Severe headache Stiff or painful neck Vomiting First-time seizure Child <6 mo or >5 yr Fever >105°C	**Do not delay treatment** Notify physician Multiple diagnostic studies or procedures Frequent consultation Continuous monitoring
●●● Level 3: Moderate Risk	**Urgent**
Earache or respiratory infection unresponsive to antibiotics History of febrile seizures or high fever spikes Signs of dehydration: sunken eyes or fontanel, dry diaper Persistent fever >102°F (>38.0°C), unresponsive to fever-reducing measures	**Refer for treatment as soon as possible** May need multiple diagnostic studies or procedures Monitor for changes in condition If vital signs abnormal, consider Level 2 Apply cooling measures
●●● Level 4: Low Risk	**Semi-Urgent**
Feeding poorly Decreased fluid intake	Reassess while waiting, per facility protocol Offer comfort measures May need simple diagnostic study or procedure

Acuity Level/Assessment	Nursing Considerations
Level 5: Lower Risk	**Non-Urgent**
Alert and oriented after a seizure Afebrile with history of febrile seizures Child wants to sleep after seizure, but easily aroused without irritability	Reassess while waiting, per facility protocol Offer comfort measures May need examination only

RELATED PROTOCOLS:

Altered Mental Status • Confusion • Diabetic Problems • Fever • Head Injury • Poisoning, Exposure or Ingestion

Notes

Sexual Assault

Acuity Level/Assessment	Nursing Considerations
●●● Level 1: Critical	**Resuscitation**
Apnea or severe respiratory distress Pulseless Unresponsive Pale, diaphoretic, and lightheaded or weak	**Refer for immediate treatment** Staff at bedside Mobilization of resuscitation team Many resources needed
●●● Level 2: High Risk	**Emergent**
Altered mental status Profuse bleeding Genital trauma Multiple traumas from assault Head injury Difficulty breathing, chest pain, or abdominal pain Suspected fractures or dislocations Victim is a minor	**Do not delay treatment** Notify physician Multiple diagnostic studies or procedures Frequent consultation Continuous monitoring
●●● Level 3: Moderate Risk	**Urgent**
Severe pain Sexual assault <72 hr previous Severe anxiety Use of objects Possible exposure to date-rape drug Abrasions, lacerations, bruising, discoloration, or swelling Victim requests examination and collection of evidence	**Refer for treatment as soon as possible** May need multiple diagnostic studies or procedures Monitor for changes in condition If vital signs abnormal, consider Level 2 Sexual assault kit and sexual assault counselor, per facility protocol

Acuity Level/Assessment	Nursing Considerations
Level 4: Low Risk	**Semi-Urgent**
Moderate pain Sexual assault >72 hr previous	Reassess while waiting, per facility protocol Offer comfort measures May need simple diagnostic study or procedure Contact sexual assault counselor, per facility protocol
Level 5: Lower Risk	Non-Urgent
Alleged assault without penetration	Reassess while waiting, per facility protocol Offer comfort measures May need examination only

RELATED PROTOCOLS:
Foreign Body, Rectum or Vagina • Rectal Problems • Vaginal Bleeding, Abnormal

Notes

Shoulder Pain

KEY QUESTIONS:
Name • Age • Onset • Allergies • Medications • Prior History • Pain Scale • Vital Signs • Oxygen Saturation • Cause

Acuity Level/Assessment	Nursing Considerations
●●● **Level 1: Critical**	**Resuscitation**
Apnea or severe respiratory distress Pulseless Unresponsive Pale, diaphoretic, and lightheaded or weak	**Refer for immediate treatment** Staff at bedside Mobilization of resuscitation team Many resources needed
●●● **Level 2: High Risk**	**Emergent**
Altered mental status Pain radiates to chest, jaw, or neck Sudden onset, no known injury, and several cardiac risk factors present Difficulty breathing Decreased circulation in affected arm Open fracture	**Do not delay treatment** Notify physician Multiple diagnostic studies or procedures Frequent consultation Continuous monitoring
●●● **Level 3: Moderate Risk**	**Urgent**
Severe pain Menstrual period >2–4 wk late and abdominal pain present Fever and swollen, red, and tender joint Inability to raise arm above head Blunt trauma Decreased sensation in the affected arm	**Refer for treatment as soon as possible** May need multiple diagnostic studies or procedures Monitor for changes in condition Check capillary refill Monitor circulation, movement, and sensation of affected extremity If vital signs abnormal, consider Level 2
●●● **Level 4: Low Risk**	**Semi-Urgent**
Moderate pain Continued pain with decreased ROM Recent injury and no improvement in pain after >3 days of ice, heat, and rest Discomfort in distal joints	Reassess while waiting, per facility protocol Offer comfort measures May need simple diagnostic study or procedure

Acuity Level/Assessment	Nursing Considerations
Level 5: Lower Risk	Non-Urgent
Chronic pain Discomfort increasing with activity Progressive joint pain and stiffness	Reassess while waiting, per facility protocol Offer comfort measures May need examination only

RELATED PROTOCOLS:

Chest Pain • Extremity Injury • Motor Vehicle Accident

Notes

Sinus Pain and Congestion

Acuity Level/Assessment	Nursing Considerations
●●● **Level 1: Critical**	**Resuscitation**
Severe respiratory distress Pale, diaphoretic, and lightheaded or weak Unresponsive Pulseless	**Refer for immediate treatment** Staff at bedside Mobilization of resuscitation team Many resources needed
●●● **Level 2: High Risk**	**Emergent**
Altered mental status Stiff neck and fever Wheezing with retractions Abnormal vital signs	**Do not delay treatment** Notify physician Multiple diagnostic studies or procedures Frequent consultation Continuous monitoring Provide IV access, per facility protocol Lab draw, per facility protocol
●●● **Level 3: Moderate Risk**	**Urgent**
Severe pain Severe headache or earache Fever >104°F (>40.0°C) and unresponsive to fever-reducing measures Mild wheezing Facial pain, swelling, redness, warmth, drainage, or fever Immunocompromised patient Fever >102°F (>39.0°C) and productive cough or shortness or breath	**Refer for treatment as soon as possible** May need multiple diagnostic studies or procedures Monitor for changes in condition If vital signs abnormal, consider Level 2
●●● **Level 4: Low Risk**	**Semi-Urgent**
Moderate pain Sore throat and persistent low-grade fever	Reassess while waiting, per facility protocol Offer comfort measures

Acuity Level/Assessment	Nursing Considerations
Level 4: Low Risk	**Semi-Urgent**
Headache worsening with movement Fever >101°F (>38.3°C) Green, brown, or yellow nasal discharge	May need simple diagnostic study or procedure
Level 5: Lower Risk	Non-Urgent
Sinus congestion Allergies Afebrile	Reassess while waiting, per facility protocol Offer comfort measures May need examination only

RELATED PROTOCOLS:
Cold Symptoms • Fever • Sore Throat

Notes

Sore Throat

Acuity Level/Assessment	Nursing Considerations
Level 1: Critical	**Resuscitation**
Severe respiratory distress Pale, diaphoretic, and lightheaded or weak O_2 saturation <90% with oxygen	**Refer for immediate treatment** Many resources needed Staff at bedside Mobilization of resuscitation team
Level 2: High Risk	**Emergent**
Altered mental status Difficulty breathing (unrelated to nasal congestion) Excessive drooling in a child Stridor or inability to swallow own saliva O_2 saturation <94% with oxygen O_2 saturation <90% on room air "Kissing tonsils" and drooling	**Do not delay treatment** Notify physician Multiple diagnostic studies or procedures Frequent consultation Constant monitoring
Level 3: Moderate Risk	**Urgent**
Severe pain and difficulty swallowing Inability to open mouth completely Signs of dehydration Sore throat and lip or mouth swelling Neck pain or rigidity History of immunosuppression, >60 yr or diabetes, and fever >100.5°F (>38.1°C) History of rheumatic fever, mitral valve prolapse, or other heart problems "Kissing tonsils" and able to swallow on saliva	**Refer for treatment as soon as possible** May need multiple diagnostic studies or procedures Monitor for changes in condition If vital signs abnormal, consider Level 2 Rapid strep test, per facility protocol

Acuity Level/Assessment	Nursing Considerations
Level 4: Low Risk	**Semi-Urgent**
Skin rash Exposure to strep throat <2 wk previous Moderate pain Hoarseness Yellow pus or white mucus at back of throat and fever Sore throat persists >3 days Earache Red or enlarged tonsils	Reassess while waiting, per facility protocol Offer comfort measures May need a simple diagnostic study or procedure Rapid strep test, per facility protocol
Level 5: Lower Risk	Non-Urgent
Mild discomfort <2 days Afebrile Chronic nasal congestion Coughing or sneezing with allergies	Reassess while waiting, per facility protocol Offer comfort measures May need examination only

RELATED PROTOCOLS:

Breathing Problems • Cold Symptoms • Cough • Ear Problems • Fever

Notes

Suicidal Behavior

KEY QUESTIONS:
Name • Age • Onset • Allergies • Prior History • Pain Scale • Vital Signs • Oxygen Saturation • Prior Suicide Attempts and Method

Acuity Level/Assessment	Nursing Considerations
●●● **Level 1: Critical**	**Resuscitation**
Apnea or severe respiratory distress Pulseless Unresponsive Pale, diaphoretic, and lightheaded or weak	**Refer for immediate treatment** Staff at bedside Mobilization of resuscitation team Many resources needed
●●● **Level 2: High Risk**	**Emergent**
Altered mental status Pulsatile bleeding from wounds Threat to self or others Overdose or poisoning Psychosis and potential harm to self or others Head trauma Hanging attempt and facial cyanosis, scleral hemorrhage, tongue swelling, petechiae Has means to carry out suicidal plan	**Do not delay treatment** Notify physician Multiple diagnostic studies or procedures Frequent consultation Continuous monitoring Apply compression dressing to control bleeding Remove and check all clothing for weapons or means to commit suicide
●●● **Level 3: Moderate Risk**	**Urgent**
Severe pain Refusal to talk, withdrawn, or no eye contact History of prior attempts Depression Intoxication Has suicidal plan with means to carry it out	**Refer for treatment as soon as possible** May need multiple diagnostic studies or procedures Maintain constant supervision of patient Monitor for changes in condition If vital signs abnormal, consider Level 2 Contact crisis personnel or social worker, per facility protocol
●●● **Level 4: Low Risk**	**Semi-Urgent**
Moderate pain Suicidal thoughts with no plans	Reassess while waiting, per facility protocol Offer comfort measures

Acuity Level/Assessment	Nursing Considerations
Level 4: Low Risk	**Semi-Urgent**
Stopped taking medication	May need simple diagnostic study or procedure Observe while waiting Contact crisis personnel or social worker, per facility protocol
Level 5: Lower Risk	Non-Urgent
History of depression controlled with medication	Reassess while waiting, per facility protocol Offer comfort measures May need examination only

RELATED PROTOCOLS:
Anxiety • Depression • Poisoning, Exposure or Ingestion

Notes

Sunburn

KEY QUESTIONS:
Name • Age • Onset • Allergies • Medications • Prior History • Severity • Pain Scale
• Vital Signs • Tetanus Immunization Status

Acuity Level/Assessment	Nursing Considerations
Level 1: Critical	**Resuscitation**
Severe respiratory distress Unresponsive Pale, diaphoretic, and lightheaded or weak Hypotension, tachycardia	**Immediate treatment** Many resources needed Staff at bedside Mobilization of resuscitation team
Level 2: High Risk	**Emergent**
Altered mental status Temperature >104.9°F (>40.5°C) and unresponsive to cooling measures Dry, hot skin and lightheadedness Diaphoresis, cool skin, and lightheadedness	**Do not delay treatment** Notify physician Multiple diagnostic studies or procedures Frequent consultation Continuous monitoring Perform cooling measures Provide IV access, per facility protocol
Level 3: Moderate Risk	**Urgent**

Severe pain
Visual changes and/or severe eye pain
Signs of dehydration
Vomiting
Circumferential burns around extremities,
   digits, or genitals
Large area of blistered skin
	Refer for treatment as soon as possible
	May need multiple diagnostic studies or
	   procedures
	Monitor for changes in condition
	If vital signs abnormal, consider Level 2

Level 4: Low Risk	**Semi-Urgent**
Moderate pain Small areas of blisters Open blisters Red streaks extending from blistered area Tetanus immunization >10 yr previous	Reassess while waiting, per facility protocol Offer comfort measures May need simple diagnostic study or procedure

Acuity Level/Assessment	Nursing Considerations
Level 5: Lower Risk	Non-Urgent
Mild sunburn Sunburn responsive to OTC analgesics	Reassess while waiting, per facility protocol May need examination only Offer comfort measures

RELATED PROTOCOLS:
Burns • Heat Exposure • Lightheadedness/Fainting

Notes

Toothache/Tooth Injury

Acuity Level/Assessment	Nursing Considerations
Level 1: Critical	**Resuscitation**
Severe respiratory distress Pale, diaphoretic, and lightheaded or weak Unresponsive Pulseless	**Immediate treatment** Many resources needed Staff at bedside Mobilization of resuscitation team
Level 2: High Risk	**Emergent**
Altered mental status Traumatic dental injuries with risk of airway compromise or neck injury Gnawing pain in lower teeth and chest, neck, shoulder, or arm Similar pain in the past and related to a heart problem Tooth knocked out Bleeding uncontrolled with constant pressure	**Do not delay treatment** Notify physician Multiple diagnostic studies or procedures Frequent consultation Continuous monitoring Tooth needs to be placed in socket ASAP; minutes count
Level 3: Moderate Risk	**Urgent**
Severe pain Facial pain, swelling, redness, warmth, drainage, or fever Fever >104°F (>40.0°C) and unresponsive to fever-reducing measures History of cardiac valve replacement Fever and neck pain Severe swelling of oral tissue	**Refer for treatment as soon as possible** May need multiple diagnostic studies or procedures Monitor for changes in condition If vital signs abnormal, consider Level 2
Level 4: Low Risk	**Semi-Urgent**
Moderate pain Swollen painful gums	Reassess while waiting, per facility protocol Offer comfort measures

Acuity Level/Assessment	Nursing Considerations
●●● **Level 4: Low Risk**	**Semi-Urgent**
Purulent drainage Foul taste or odor in mouth Recent dental work in painful area Chipped or fractured tooth	May need simple diagnostic study or procedure
●●● Level 5: Lower Risk	Non-Urgent
Sores in mouth Loose or decayed tooth Sensitive to heat, cold, or pressure Tooth discolored	Reassess while waiting, per facility protocol May need examination only Offer comfort measures

RELATED PROTOCOLS:
Mouth Problems

Notes

Urinary Catheter Problems

KEY QUESTIONS:

Name • Age • Onset • Allergies • Medications • Prior History • Severity • Pain Scale • Vital Signs • Date Catheter Inserted

Acuity Level/Assessment	Nursing Considerations
Level 1: Critical	**Resuscitation**
Severe respiratory distress Pale, diaphoretic, and lightheaded or weak Pulseless Unresponsive	**Refer for immediate treatment** Staff at bedside Mobilization of resuscitation team Many resources needed
Level 2: High Risk	**Emergent**
Altered mental status Severe flank, abdominal, or back pain and fever >102°F (>39.0°C) Profuse bright red blood from catheter	**Do not delay treatment** Notify physician Multiple diagnostic studies or procedures Frequent consultation Continuous monitoring
Level 3: Moderate Risk	**Urgent**
Severe pain Gross hematuria Passing clots through catheter Painful, distended bladder No urine output >8 hr Surgically placed catheter or tube displaced	**Refer for treatment as soon as possible** May need multiple diagnostic studies or procedures Monitor for changes in condition If vital signs abnormal, consider Level 2
Level 4: Low Risk	**Semi-Urgent**
Moderate pain Recent urological surgery Taking a blood-thinning agent and urine pink or red Skin irritation near meatus Cloudy, foul-smelling urine Fever >100.4°F (>38.0°C)	Reassess while waiting, per facility protocol Offer comfort measures May need simple diagnostic study or procedure

Acuity Level/Assessment	Nursing Considerations
Level 5: Lower Risk	Non-Urgent
Catheter leak Mild discomfort	Reassess while waiting, per facility protocol Offer comfort measures May need examination only

RELATED PROTOCOLS:
Abdominal Pain, Adult • Abdominal Pain, Pediatric • Fever • Urination Problems

Notes

Urination Problems

KEY QUESTIONS:

Name • Age • Onset • Allergies • Medications • Prior History • Severity • Pain Scale • Vital Signs

Acuity Level/Assessment	Nursing Considerations
●●● Level 1: Critical	**Resuscitation**
Severe respiratory distress Pale, diaphoretic, and lightheaded or weak Pulseless Unresponsive	**Refer for immediate treatment** Staff at bedside Mobilization of resuscitation team Many resources needed
●●● Level 2: High Risk	**Emergent**
Altered mental status Severe abdominal pain with fever >102°F (>39.0°C) Hematuria and flank trauma, history of renal transplant, or severe abdominal or flank pain Severe abdominal pain and unable to void >8 hr or catheter bag empty >8 hr Traumatic injury to urethra and unable to stop bleeding with pressure	**Do not delay treatment** Notify physician Multiple diagnostic studies or procedures Frequent consultation Continuous monitoring
●●● Level 3: Moderate Risk	**Urgent**
Severe pain Fever >102°F (>39.0°C) Persistent flank, back, or abdominal pain Hematuria and colicky flank pain or use of anticoagulants Pain with urination, back or flank pain, and fever >100.5°F (>38.1°C) Pain or bleeding and history of diabetes or immunosuppression New onset of incontinence History of renal or prostate disease Recent trauma (back, abdominal, genital area)	**Refer for treatment as soon as possible** May need multiple diagnostic studies or procedures Monitor for changes in condition If vital signs abnormal, consider Level 2 Urine sample and dip, per facility protocol

Acuity Level/Assessment	Nursing Considerations
●●● **Level 3: Moderate Risk**	**Urgent**
Unable to urinate >4–8 hr Recent urinary or abdominal surgery and 　dysuria	
●●● **Level 4: Low Risk**	**Semi-Urgent**
Moderate pain Fever >100.4°F (>38.0°C) Nausea or vomiting Genital herpes or STD Difficulty urinating after sexual intercourse Urinary frequency, urgency, and/or hematuria Full bladder and unable to urinate <4 hr	Reassess while waiting, per facility protocol Offer comfort measures May need simple diagnostic study or procedure Urine sample and dip, per facility protocol
●●● Level 5: Lower Risk	Non-Urgent
Burning sensation after exposure to bubble 　baths, nylon underwear, soaps, or other 　products applied to the perineal area Urinary frequency or fullness Nocturia	Reassess while waiting, per facility protocol Offer comfort measures May need examination only

RELATED PROTOCOLS:

Abdominal Pain, Adult • Abdominal Pain, Pediatric • Back Pain • Fever • Urinary Catheter Problems

Notes

Vaginal Bleeding, Abnormal

KEY QUESTIONS:
Name • Age • Onset • Allergies • Medications • Prior History • Severity • Pain Scale
• Vital Signs • Birth Control Measures • Last Menstrual Period • Number of Pregnancies

Acuity Level/Assessment	Nursing Considerations
Level 1: Critical	**Resuscitation**
Severe respiratory distress Pale, diaphoretic, and lightheaded or weak Pulseless Unresponsive	**Refer for immediate treatment** Staff at bedside Mobilization of resuscitation team Many resources needed
Level 2: High Risk	**Emergent**

Altered mental status
Sexual assault and profuse bleeding or injury
   with an object
Profuse bleeding >3 full-size pad/hr
Passing products of conception
Diaphoretic
History of blood disorders
Pregnancy >20 wk
Hypotension
Vaginal bleeding, abdominal or shoulder pain,
   last period 2–4 wk late and possibility of
   pregnancy
Retained foreign object
	Do not delay treatment
	Notify physician
	Multiple diagnostic studies or procedures
	Frequent consultation
	Continuous monitoring

Level 3: Moderate Risk	**Urgent**

Severe pain
Nausea, vomiting, or lightheadedness
Increased thirst or signs of dehydration
Increased abdominal pain with movement
Orthostatic changes
Recent abortion or miscarriage with fever,
   pain, and increasing bleeding
	Refer for treatment as soon as possible
	May need multiple diagnostic studies or
	   procedures
	Monitor for changes in condition
	If vital signs abnormal, consider Level 2
	Measure orthostatic vital signs

Acuity Level/Assessment	Nursing Considerations
Level 4: Low Risk	**Semi-Urgent**
Moderate pain Cramping Heavier-than-normal period Bleeding increased with increase in activity or change in birth control pills Bleeding >10 days	Reassess while waiting, per facility protocol Offer comfort measures May need simple diagnostic study or procedure
Level 5: Lower Risk	Non-Urgent
Spotty bleeding after sexual intercourse Recently started taking oral contraceptives Normal menses Patient concerned about menopause or pregnancy	Reassess while waiting, per facility protocol Offer comfort measures May need examination only

RELATED PROTOCOLS:

Foreign Body, Rectum or Vagina • Pregnancy, Vaginal Discharge

Notes

Vomiting

KEY QUESTIONS:

Name • Age • Onset • Allergies • Medications • Prior History • Severity • Pain Scale • Vital Signs • Health of Other Household Members • Recent Trauma

Acuity Level/Assessment	Nursing Considerations
● ● ● Level 1: Critical	**Resuscitation**
Severe respiratory distress Pale, diaphoretic, and lightheaded or weak Unresponsive Pulseless	**Refer for immediate treatment** Staff at bedside Mobilization of resuscitation team Many resources needed
● ● ● Level 2: High Risk	**Emergent**
Altered mental status Head injury Persistent vomiting of frank blood or coffee grounds–like emesis Chest, jaw, or arm pain Abdominal trauma Diabetic and glucose >400 mg/dL	**Do not delay treatment** Notify physician Multiple diagnostic studies or procedures Frequent consultation Continuous monitoring
● ● ● Level 3: Moderate Risk	**Urgent**
Severe abdominal pain or headache >2 hr Signs of dehydration Possible ingestion of, or exposure to poisonous substance History of diabetes, cancer, other chronic illness, or immunosuppression Age >60 yr and vomited more than once Fever >104°F (>40°C) Orthostatic vital signs	**Refer for treatment as soon as possible** May need multiple diagnostic studies or procedures Monitor for changes in condition If abnormal vital signs, consider Level 2

Acuity Level/Assessment	Nursing Considerations
Level 4: Low Risk	**Semi-Urgent**
Moderate pain Recent ingestion of an antibiotic, pain medication, or new medication Vomiting >48 hr	Reassess while waiting, per facility protocol Offer comfort measures May need a simple diagnostic study or procedure
Level 5: Lower Risk	Non-Urgent
Vomiting <24 hr Recent surgery, hospitalization, or diagnostic procedure Other household members are ill Excessive ingestion of food, alcohol, or fluids Possible pregnancy	Reassess while waiting, per facility protocol Offer comfort measures May need an examination only

RELATED PROTOCOLS:
Abdominal Pain, Adult • Abdominal Pain, Pediatric • Diarrhea, Adult • Diarrhea, Pediatric • Fever • Head Injury • Poisoning, Exposure or Ingestion • Pregnancy, Vomiting

Notes

Weakness

KEY QUESTIONS:
Name • Age • Onset • Allergies • Medications • Prior History • Severity • Vital Signs • Oxygen Saturation • Pain Scale (for chest pain, see Chest Pain; for difficulty breathing, see Breathing Problems; for altered mental status, see Altered Mental Status)

Acuity Level/Assessment	Nursing Considerations
●●● **Level 1: Critical**	**Resuscitation**
Apnea or severe respiratory distress Unresponsive Pale, diaphoretic, and lightheaded or weak Pulseless	**Refer for immediate treatment** Staff at bedside Mobilization of resuscitation team Many resources needed
●●● **Level 2: High Risk**	**Emergent**
Sudden onset or persistent altered mental status Drug or alcohol overdose Inability to stand, walk, or bear weight Severe headache Chest pain Rapid heartbeat with syncope/diaphoresis Sudden onset of weakness to one side of the body Weakness in face, arm, or leg Visual disturbances Speech and language problems Irregular pulse Severe abdominal pain Loss of movement in arms or legs, confusion, difficulty speaking, numbness, tingling or blurred vision, and onset <2 hr Hand or foot cold or blue Headache, fever, and stiff or painful neck Orthostatic vital signs	**Do not delay treatment** Notify physician Multiple diagnostic studies or procedures Frequent consultation Continuous monitoring Finger-stick glucose

Acuity Level/Assessment	Nursing Considerations
● ● ● Level 3: Moderate Risk	**Urgent**
Recent head injury or trauma (rule out head bleed) Persistent high fever Severe abdominal pain and normal vital signs Temporary slurred speech or weakened grips Pain, swelling, warmth, or redness in affected limb Severe pain interfering with normal activity	**Refer for treatment as soon as possible** May need multiple diagnostic studies or procedures Monitor for changes in condition If vital signs abnormal, consider Level 2
● ● ● Level 4: Low Risk	**Semi-Urgent**
History of dieting or use of diuretics Gradual onset of numbness, tingling, or burning sensation in extremities Pain radiates to arm or leg Fever; cough; green, yellow, or brown sputum; body aches for >24 hr; and unresponsive to home care measures History of taking cholesterol-lowering medication Recent history of frequent falls	Offer comfort measures Reassess while waiting, per facility protocol May need a simple diagnostic study or procedure
● ● ● Level 5: Lower Risk	Non-Urgent
Exhaustion Occasional weakness History of neuromuscular problems that are unresponsive to medication Increased exercise, activity level, or stress History of muscular pain	Offer comfort measures Reassess while waiting, per facility protocol May need examination only

RELATED PROTOCOLS:
Altered Mental Status • Breathing Problems • Chest Pain • Fever • Headache

Wound Infection

KEY QUESTIONS:
Name • Age • Onset • Allergies • Medications • Prior History • Severity • Pain Scale • Vital Signs

Acuity Level/Assessment	Nursing Considerations
●●● **Level 1: Critical**	**Resuscitation**
Severe respiratory distress Pale, diaphoretic, and lightheaded or weak Unresponsive Pulseless	**Refer for immediate treatment** Staff at bedside Mobilization of resuscitation team Many resources needed
●●● **Level 2: High Risk**	**Emergent**
Altered mental status Sutured or stapled wound >50% open	**Do not delay treatment** Notify physician Multiple diagnostic studies or procedures Frequent consultation Continuous monitoring
●●● **Level 3: Moderate Risk**	**Urgent**
Severe pain Surgical wound dehiscence Purulent drainage Fever Swollen lymph nodes Red streaking away from the wound Headache or general illness	**Refer for treatment as soon as possible** May need multiple diagnostic studies or procedures Monitor for changes in condition If abnormal vital signs, consider Level 2
●●● **Level 4: Low Risk**	**Semi-Urgent**

Moderate pain
High-risk history (e.g., diabetes,
  immunosuppression, chronic illness,
  chemotherapy, use of steroids) and wound
  not healing well
	Reassess while waiting, per facility protocol
	Offer comfort measures
	May need a simple diagnostic study or
	  procedure

Acuity Level/Assessment	Nursing Considerations
●●● Level 5: Lower Risk	Non-Urgent
Wound itching Tetanus immunization >5–10 yr previous	Reassess while waiting, per facility protocol Offer comfort measures May need an examination only

RELATED PROTOCOLS:
Abdominal Pain, Adult • Abdominal Pain, Pediatric • Diabetic Problems

Notes

Wrist Pain and Swelling

Name • Age • Onset • Allergies • Medications • Prior History • Severity • Pain Scale • Vital Signs • Mechanism of Injury

Acuity Level/Assessment	Nursing Considerations
Level 1: Critical	**Resuscitation**
Severe respiratory distress Pale, diaphoretic, and lightheaded or weak Unresponsive	**Refer for immediate treatment** Staff at bedside Mobilization of resuscitation team Many resources needed
Level 2: High Risk	**Emergent**
Altered mental status Pulsatile bleeding No radial pulse Cyanosis of the hand Open fracture Suicidal behavior	**Do not delay treatment** Notify physician Multiple diagnostic studies or procedures Frequent consultation Continuous monitoring Continuous observation of suicidal patient
Level 3: Moderate Risk	**Urgent**
Severe pain Unsplinted angulated deformity Wrist swollen to twice its normal size Fever, drainage, red streaks	**Refer for treatment as soon as possible** May need multiple diagnostic studies or procedures Monitor for changes in condition If abnormal vital signs, consider Level 2
Level 4: Low Risk	**Semi-Urgent**
Moderate pain Splinted deformity High-risk mechanism of injury Decreased mobility Inability to make a fist	Reassess while waiting, per facility protocol Offer comfort measures May need a simple diagnostic study or procedure

Acuity Level/Assessment	Nursing Considerations
Level 5: Lower Risk	Non-Urgent
Pain, swelling, or discoloration Chronic discomfort (old injury) History of arthritis or tendonitis Pain increasing with repetitive activities	Reassess while waiting, per facility protocol Offer comfort measures May need an examination only

RELATED PROTOCOLS:
Extremity Injury • Motor Vehicle Accident • Shoulder Pain

Notes

Bibliography

Anscombe Wood, D. (2004, June 7). On the level(s). *NurseWeek*. Available at: http://www.nurseweek.com news/features/04-06/triage.asp. Accessed April 26, 2005.

Beckstrand, R. L., & Sanders, E. K. (2003). A 39-year-old man with left shoulder pain: Comparing 3- and 5-point triage scales. *Journal of Emergency Nursing, 29*(4), 387–389.

Bowman, M., & Baxt, W. (2003). *Office emergencies.* Philadelphia: Saunders.

Briggs, J. (2002). *Telephone triage protocols for nurses* (2nd ed.). Philadelphia: Lippincott Williams & Wilkins.

Dart, R. (2000). *The 5-minute toxicology consult.* Philadelphia: Lippincott Williams & Wilkins.

Davis, M. A., Greenough, G., & Votey, S. (Eds.) (1999). *Signs & symptoms in emergency medicine.* St. Louis: Mosby.

Emde, K. (2003). MDMA (Ecstasy) in the emergency department. *Journal of Emergency Nursing, 29*(5), 440–443.

Ferri, F. (2003). *Ferri's clinical advisor: Instant diagnosis and treatment.* St. Louis: Mosby.

Grossman, V. G. A. (2003). *Quick reference to triage* (2nd ed.). Philadelphia: Lippincott Williams & Wilkins.

Molczan, K. (2001). Triaging orthopedic injuries. *Journal of Emergency Nursing, 27*(3), 297–300.

Muller, A. A. (2003). Small amounts of some drugs can be toxic to young children: One pill or one swallow can require aggressive treatment. *Journal of Emergency Nursing, 29*(3), 290–293.

Rosen, P., Barkin, R., Hayden, R., Schaider, J., & Wolfe, R. (1999). *The 5-minute emergency medicine consult.* Philadelphia: Lippincott Williams & Wilkins.

RnCeus.com (2002). Biochemical terrorism: An ER resource. Available at: http://www.rnceus.com. Accessed April 26, 2005.

Tipsord-Klinkhammer, B. (Ed.) (1998). *Triage: Meeting the challenge* (2nd ed.). Des Plaines, IL: Emergency Nurses Association.

Travers, D., Waller, A., Bowling, M., Flowers, D., & Tintinalli, J. (2002). Five-level triage system more effective than three-level in tertiary emergency department. *Journal of Emergency Nursing 28*(5), 395–400.

Zimmermann, P. G. (2003). Orienting ED nurses to triage: Using scenario-based test-style questions to promote critical thinking. *Journal of Emergency Nursing, 29*(3), 256–258.

Zimmermann, P. G. (2003). Tricks for the ED trade. *Journal of Emergency Nursing, 29*(5), 453–458.

The PQRSTT Mnemonic Assessment Guide

P = Provoking factors
- What makes it (pain, breathing, etc.) worse?
- What makes it better?
- Any known trauma or injury?

Q = Quality of pain
- What does it feel like?
- Does the patient use descriptive words, such as burning, stabbing, crushing, or tearing?

R = Region/Radiation
- Where is the pain?
- Is it in one spot?
- Does it start in one spot and travel to another?
- Ask the patient to point to where it hurts using one finger.

S = Severity of pain
- If the patient were to describe the pain with a number from 0 to 10, with 0 being the least severe and 10 being the worst pain imaginable, what number would the patient give this pain?

T = Time
- When did this start?
- How long have the symptoms persisted?
- How long did it last?
- Has it ever happened before?

T = Treatment
- Has the patient taken any medication to treat this?
- What time was the last dose?
- Has the patient done anything to treat him- or herself?
- What has or has not worked for the patient?

Appendix B

Pediatric Vital Signs: Normal Ranges

Age Group	Respiratory Rate	Heart Rate	Systolic Blood Pressure	Weight Kilogram	Weight Pounds
Newborn	30–50	120–160	50–70	2–3	4.5–7
Infant (1–12 mo)	20–30	80–140	70–100	4–10	9–22
Toddler (1–3 yr)	20–30	80–130	80–110	10–14	22–31
Preschooler (3–5 yr)	20–30	80–120	80–110	14–18	31–40
School Age (6–12 yr)	18–25	70–110	85–120	20–42	41–92
Adolescent (13+ yr)	12–20	55–110	100–120	>50	>110

REMEMBER:
- The patient's normal range should always be taken into consideration.
- Heart rate, blood pressure, and respiratory rate are expected to increase during times of fever or stress.
- Respiratory rate on infants should be counted for a full 60 seconds.
- In a clinically decompensating child, the blood pressure will be the last to change. Just because your pediatric patient's blood pressure is normal, don't assume that your patient is stable.
- Bradycardia in children is an ominous sign, usually a result of hypoxia. Act quickly, as this child is extremely critical.

Appendix C

Ibuprofen Dosage Chart*

Approximate Weight Range (kg)	Approximate Weight Range (lb)	Dose (mg)	Dosage				
			Drops (50 mg/ 1.25 mL)	Syrup (100 mg/ 5 mL)	Chewable (50 mg)	Junior Tablets (100 mg)	Adult Tablets (200 mg)
2.5	5.5	25	0.625 mL	—	—	—	—
2.6–5	5.7–11	50	1.25 mL	2.5 mL	1 tab	—	—
5–7.5	11–16.5	75	1.875 mL	3.75 mL	1.5 tabs	—	—
7.6–10	16.7–22	100	2.5 mL	5.0 mL	2 tabs	1 tab	—
11–12	24–26	125	3 mL	6.25 mL	2.5 tabs	—	—
13–15	28–33	150	3.75 mL	7.5 mL	3 tabs	1.5 tabs	—
16–17	35–37	175	—	8.75 mL	3.5 tabs	—	—
18–20	39–44	200	—	10 mL	4 tabs	2 tabs	1 tab
21–25	46–55	250	—	12.5 mL	5 tabs	2.5 tabs	—
26–30	57–66	300	—	15 mL	6 tabs	3 tabs	1.5 tabs
31–35	68–77	350	—	17.5 mL	7 tabs	3.5 tabs	—
36–40	79–88	400	—	20 mL	8 tabs	4 tabs	2 tabs
41–45	90–99	450	—	—	—	4.5 tabs	—
46–50	101–110	500	—	—	—	5 tabs	2.5 tabs
51–55	112–121	550	—	—	—	5.5 tabs	—
>56–60	>123–132	600	—	—	—	6 tabs	3 tabs

*Do not use Ibuprofen in children less than 6 months of age or those with chickenpox.

Appendix D

Acetaminophen Dosage Chart

Approximate Weight Range (kg)	Approximate Weight Range (lb)	Dose (mg)	Dosage				
			Drops (80 mg/ 0.8 mL)	Syrup (160 mg/ mL)	Chewable (80 mg)	Chewable (160 mg)	Adult Tablets (325 mg)
<5.9	<13	40	1/2 dropper (0.4 mL)	1.25 mL	—	—	—
5.9–9	13–20	80	1 dropper (0.8 mL)	2.5 mL	—	—	—
9–11	21–26	120	1 1/2 dropper (1.2 mL)	3.75 mL	—	—	—
12–15	27–35	160	2 droppers (1.6 mL)	5 mL	2 tabs	—	—
16–19	36–43	240	3 droppers (2.4 mL)	7.5 mL	3 tabs	1.5 tabs	—
20–28	44–62	320	—	10 mL	4 tabs	2 tabs	1 tab
28–35	63–79	400	—	12.5 mL	5 tabs	2.5 tabs	—
36–40	80–89	480	—	15 mL	6 tabs	3 tabs	—
41–45	90–99	560	—	17.5 mL	7 tabs	3.5 tabs	—
46–50	101–110	650	—	20 mL	—	4 tabs	2 tabs
51–55	112–121	825	—	25 mL	—	5 tabs	—
56–60	123–132	900	—	28 mL	—	5.5 tabs	—
61–65	133–143	975	—	30 mL	—	6 tabs	3 tabs
>65	>143						

Temperature Conversion Chart

Celsius	Fahrenheit
43.0	109.4
42.0	107.6
41.0	105.8
40.5	104.9
40.0	104.0
39.5	103.1
39.0	102.2
38.5	101.3
38.0	100.4
37.5	99.5
37.0	98.6
36.5	97.7
36.0	96.8
35.0	95.0
34.0	93.2
33.0	91.4
32.0	89.6
31.0	87.8
30.0	86.0
29.0	84.2
28.0	82.4
27.0	80.6
26.0	78.8
25.0	77.0
24.0	75.2
23.0	73.4

(*continued*)

Celsius	Fahrenheit
22.0	71.6
21.0	69.8
20.0	68.0
19.0	66.2
18.0	64.4

Formula for Fahrenheit to Celsius: (1.8 × Celsius reading) + 32

Formula for Celsius to Fahrenheit: 0.55 × (Fahrenheit reading − 32)

Weight Conversion Chart

Pound	Kilogram
1	0.45
2	0.90
3	1.35
4	1.80
5	2.25
6	2.70
8	3.60
10	4.50
11	5
22	10
33	15
44	20
55	25
66	30
77	35
88	40
99	45
110	50
121	55
132	60
143	65
154	70
165	75
176	80
187	85
198	90
209	95

(continued)

Pound	Kilogram
220	100
231	105
242	110
253	115
264	120
275	125
286	130
297	135

Differential Diagnosis of Abdominal Pain

Possible Diagnosis	Signs and Symptoms
Abdominal Aortic Aneurysm	Asymptomatic until leakage or rupture occurs
	Abrupt onset of severe back, flank, or abdominal pain
	Pulsatile abdominal mass, mottling of lower extremities, signs of shock
Appendicitis	Diffuse pain in epigastric or periumbilical area for 1–2 days
	Localization of pain over the right lower quadrant between the umbilicus and right iliac crest
	Anorexia, nausea/vomiting, fever, tachycardia, pallor, peritoneal signs
	Increased pain with stairs, walking, etc.
Bowel Obstruction	Severe, crampy, colicky abdominal pain
	Vomiting, constipation, hypotension, tachycardia, abdominal distention, hyperactive bowel sounds, fever
Cholecystitis (Inflammation of Gallbladder)	Colicky discomfort in the right upper quadrant mid-epigastric area
	Pain radiating to the shoulders and back
	Nausea/vomiting, fever, tachycardia, tachypnea, abdominal guarding, jaundice, malaise
Cholelithiasis (Presence of Gallbladder Stones)	Severe, steady, or colicky pain in the upper abdominal quadrant, often right-sided
	Pain usually begins 3–6 hours after a large meal
	Pain radiation to scapula, back, or right shoulder
	Nausea, vomiting, dyspepsia, mild to moderate jaundice
Constipation/Fecal Impaction	Clinically defined as defecation <3 times per week
	Each patient may interpret the symptoms differently
	Fatigue, abdominal discomfort, headache, low back pain, anorexia, restlessness
Duodenal or Ileojejunal Hematoma	Caused by a blow to the abdomen
	Immediate bruising over upper quadrant of abdomen
Epididymitis	Infection or inflammation of the epididymis

(*continued*)

Possible Diagnosis	Signs and Symptoms
	Swelling and enlargement of the epididymis, sudden swelling of the spermatic cord, fever, dysuria, urethral discharge
Intussusception	Paroxysms of acute abdominal pain, intermittent with pain-free episodes
	Currant jelly, mucus-type stools or rectal bleeding
	Fever, lethargy, vomiting (food, mucus, fecal matter), dehydration
Orchitis	Inflammation or infection of the testicle
	Intense pain and swelling of the scrotum, dysuria, urethral discharge, fever, discomfort in the groin/lower abdomen, acute illness
Pancreatitis	Severe, constant, upper quadrant midepigastric pain that radiates to the midback
	Pain worsens when lying flat on back, relieved when lying on side with knees drawn up
	Nausea, vomiting, fever, pallor, hypotension, tachycardia, tachypnea, restlessness, malaise, fatty or foul-smelling stools, abdominal distention, pulmonary crackles
Peritonitis	Severe pain that gradually increases in intensity and worsens with movement
	Riding in car, climbing stairs, or jumping on one foot greatly worsens pain
	Radiation of pain to shoulder, back, or chest
	Nausea, vomiting, fever, abdominal distention, rigidity, and tenderness
Renal Calculi	Location of stone depicts associated pain: flank, lower abdominal quadrant, low back, groin, testicular, labial, or urethral meatus
	Pain radiation varies on stone location
	Nausea, vomiting, pallor, diaphoresis, marked restlessness, dehydration
Ruptured Ovarian Cyst	Sudden, severe, unilateral lower quadrant abdominal pain associated with exercise or intercourse
	Delayed or prolonged menstruation, vomiting, ascites, signs of peritonitis
Tubal Pregnancy	Intermittent diffuse abdominal pain
	Radiation of pain to shoulder
	Vaginal spotting/bleeding, syncope, dizziness, signs of peritonitis or shock
Urinary Tract Infection	Lower quadrant abdominal or pelvic pain
	Urinary burning, frequency, urgency, hematuria, foul smelling urine, fever, bladder spasms
Cystitis	Dysuria, urinary frequency and urgency, fever, hematuria
Pyelonephritis	Flank or back pain
	Urinary frequency, dysuria, fever, malaise, nausea, vomiting, chills

(continued)

Possible Diagnosis	Signs and Symptoms
Prostatitis	Perineal aching, low back pain
	Urinary frequency, dysuria, fever, malaise, urethral discharge, prostate swelling
Testicular Torsion	Sudden onset of severe, unilateral testicular pain and tenderness
	Nausea, vomiting, fever, scrotal mass
Ulcer (Gastric, Duodenal, Esophageal)	Colicky, burning, squeezing pain in the epigastric or midback area
	Pain intensity is variable, often begins 1–3 hr after meals, worsens at night
	Nausea, vomiting, hematemesis, abdominal guarding, decreased or absent bowel sounds

Appendix H

Differential Diagnosis of Chest Pain

System	Cause	Characteristics
Cardiovascular	Acute Myocardial Infarction	Pain may be described as aching, pressing, squeezing, burning, tight Intensity: vague to severe Location of pain may be substernal, epigastric, or between the shoulder blades Pain may radiate to the neck, jaw, arm, back Women may describe symptoms more of nausea, fatigue, shortness of breath Diabetic neuropathy patients may have only vague pain
	Aneurysm	Pain may be described as searing, continuous, severe Pain may radiate to the back, neck, or shoulder(s) Associated signs and symptoms: hypotension, diaphoresis, syncope
	Angina	Pain may be described as squeezing, pressing, tight, relieved with rest or nitroglycerin Pain may be persistent and intermittent Occurs with activity, anxiety, sex, heavy meals, smoking, or at rest Associated signs and symptoms: dyspnea, nausea, vomiting, diaphoresis, indigestion
	Cardiac Contusion	Cardiac compression between the sternum and vertebral column (falls, MVAs, blunt chest trauma, etc.) May have EKG changes such as right bundle branch block, ST-T wave abnormalities, Q waves, atrial fibrillation, premature ventricular contractions, and A-V conduction disturbances
	Heart Transplant	REJECTION may present with low-grade fever, fatigue, dyspnea, peripheral edema, pulmonary crackles, malaise, pericardial friction rub, arrhythmias, decreased EKG voltage, hypotension, increased jugular distention

(continued)

System	Cause	Characteristics
	Pericarditis	**INFECTION** may be masked by use of immunosuppressive therapy; look for low-grade fever, cough, and malaise
		CORONARY HEART DISEASE is common in patients with heart transplants
		Pain may be described as severe, continuous, worse when lying on left side
		Radiation of pain to shoulder or neck
		History may include recent cardiac surgery, viral illness, or myocardial infarction
		Diffuse ST elevation in multiple leads
		PQ segment depression
	Tachydysrhythmias	Pain may be described as severe, crushing, or generalized over chest
		Associated signs and symptoms: anxiety, tachycardia, dizziness, impending doom
Gastrointestinal	Hiatal Hernia	Pain may be described as sharp, over the epigastrium
		Occurs with heavy meals, bending over, lying down
	Gastroesophageal Reflux Disease (GERD)	Pain may be described as burning, heartburn, pressing
		Nonradiating pain, not influenced by activity
Musculo-skeletal	Costochondritis	Pain may be described as sharp or severe
		Localized to affected area with tenderness on palpation
		Associated signs and symptoms: cough, "cold"
	Muscle Strain	Pain may be described as aching
		Occurs with increased use or exercise of upper-body muscles
		Pain is severe, with localization over area of trauma
		Pain worsens with palpations, movement, or cough
		May have dyspnea
Pulmonary	Noxious Fumes/ Smoke Inhalation	Pain may be described as searing; sense of suffocation
		History includes exposure to fire, pesticide, carbon monoxide, paint, chemicals
		Associated signs and symptoms: dyspnea, hypoxia, cough, pallor, ashen skin, cyanosis, singed nasal hairs, soot in oropharynx, gray or black sputum, hoarseness, drooling
		Those with carbon monoxide poisoning may additionally show nausea, headache, confusion, dizziness, irritability, decreased judgment, ataxia, collapse
	Pleural Effusion	Pain may be described as sharp, localized, gradual onset, yet continuous
		Dyspnea on exertion or at rest
		Pain worsens with breathing, coughing, movement
		Common in smokers

(*continued*)

System	Cause	Characteristics
Pulmonary	**Pneumonia**	Pain may be described as continuous, dull discomfort to severe pain
		Associated signs and symptoms: fever, shortness of breath, tachycardia, malaise, cough, tachypnea
		Children may complain of abdominal pain instead of chest pain
	Pneumothorax	Pain may be described as sudden onset, sharp, severe
		Associated signs and symptoms: shortness of breath
	Pulmonary Embolism	Acute shortness of breath
		Risk factors include recent long bone fractures, surgery, smoking, use of oral contraceptives, sitting for long periods of time (e.g., long air travel)
Other	**Anxiety**	Pain may be described as aching, stabbing
		Associated with stressful event, anxiety
		Associated signs and symptoms: hyperventilation, carpal spasms, palpitations, weakness, fear, sense of impending doom

Source: Grossman, V. A. (2003). *Quick Reference to Triage* (2nd ed.). Philadelphia: Lippincott Williams & Wilkins.

Headache: Common Characteristics

Headache Type	Characteristics

Cerebellar Hemorrhage	Pain:
	  Moderate to severe
	Associated signs and symptoms:
	  Confusion
	  Vomiting
	  Altered gait

Cluster Headaches	Pain:
	  Very painful
	  Knifelike
	  Unilateral
	  Over the eye
	Associated signs and symptoms:
	  Excessive tearing
	  Facial swelling
	  Redness of the eye
	  Diaphoresis

Increased Intracranial Pressure	Pain:
	  Usually not excruciating
	Associated symptoms:
	  Nausea or vomiting
	  Lethargy
	  Diplopia
	  Transient visual difficulty

Meningitis	Pain:
	  Mild to severe
	  Neck pain or stiffness
	Associated signs and symptoms:
	  Fever
	  Malaise
	  Decreased appetite
	  Irritability

(*continued*)

Headache Type	Characteristics

Migraines	Pain:
	  Periodic with gradual onset
	  Throbbing, severe
	  Frequently unilateral, may progress to bilateral
	  Often above the eye(s)
	Associated signs and symptoms:
	  Photophobia
	  Sensitivity to sound
	  Nausea
	  Vomiting

Sinus Headache	Pain:
	  Over the sinus areas (above the eyes, beside the nose, or over the cheekbone)
	Associated signs and symptoms:
	  Fever
	  Nasal drainage or congestion
	  Ear pain
	  Tenderness, swelling, or erythema of the sinus area

Subarachnoid Hemorrhage	Pain:
	  "Worst headache of my life"
	Associated signs and symptoms:
	  With or without transient impairment of consciousness

Tension	Pain:
	  Diffuse yet steady dull pain or pressure
	  "Band-like" (back of head and neck, across forehead, and/or temporal areas)

MVA Triage Questions

When did the accident occur?
- Day
- Time

Where did it occur?
- Highway
- Country road
- City street
- Off road
- Speedway

Was the patient wearing a seat belt?
- What type? (lap, shoulder, etc.)
- Effectiveness during the accident?

What speed was the patient's car traveling?
- Approximate speed of other vehicles involved in accident
- Approximate speed of patient's vehicle

Where was the patient sitting in the car?
- Driver
- Front seat passenger
- Back seat passenger
- Box of the truck

What kind of vehicle was the patient in?

What damage was done to the vehicle?
- Sport utility vehicle
- Compact car
- Other motorized vehicle
- Motorcycle

(continued)

Did the airbag deploy?

Did the patient lose consciousness?
- For how long?

What is the last thing the patient remembers *before* the accident?

What is the first thing the patient remembers *after* the accident?

How was the patient injured in the car?
- Flying objects within the car
- Car crushed by other vehicle, tree, pole, etc.

Was the patient thrown from the car?
- Was something in the car thrown against the patient?

Was the patient ambulatory at the scene?
- Did the patient need to be extricated from the vehicle?
- How long did it take?

Were there any other people in the car?
- Were they injured?
- What are their injuries?

Was the pediatric patient in a car seat?
- Where was the car seat located within the vehicle?
- Was it struck by a deployed air bag?
- Was the car seat strapped tightly with the seatbelt?

Were there law enforcement personnel at the scene?
- If so, which agency?

Does the patient wear:
- Contact lenses?
- Glasses?
- Hearing aid?
- Were they worn at the scene?
- Dentures?
- Female patients: Is a tampon in place?
- Insulin pump or other medical device? Pacemaker? Internal cardiac defibrillator?

Where is the patient experiencing pain?

Is the patient taking any medication, especially aspirin or other anticoagulants?

Is there anyone the patient wishes to have notified?

Mechanisms of Injury from Trauma: Adult

Trauma	Associated Injuries
Pedestrian struck by car • Adult point of impact is usually knee/hip	Fractures of the femur, tibia, and fibula on side of impact Fractured pelvis Contralateral ligament damage to knee
Pedestrian struck by car • Short adult/child point of impact involves chest and/or head	Contralateral skull fracture Chest injury with rib and/or sternal fracture May be thrown, resulting in head/back injury Shoulder dislocation and/or scapular fracture Patellar and lower femur fracture
Pedestrian dragged under a vehicle	Pelvic fracture
MVA: Unrestrained front seat passenger • Front impact	Posterior dislocation of acetabulum Fractures of femurs and/or patellas
MVA: Unrestrained driver • Front impact	Head injury, c-spine injury, pelvic fracture Flail chest, fractured sternum Aortic or tracheal tears Pulmonary/cardiac contusion Ruptured or lacerated liver or spleen Femur and/or patellar fracture, hip dislocation
MVA: Unrestrained driver or passenger • Side impact	Chest: flail, fractured sternum, pulmonary/cardiac contusion Fractures of clavicle, acetabulum, pelvis Lateral neck strain or injury Driver: ruptured spleen Passenger: ruptured liver
MVA: Passenger without headrest restraint • Rear impact	Hyperextension of neck resulting in high c-spine or vertebral fracture or ruptured disk(s), causing intradural hemorrhage, edema, spinal cord compression

(continued)

Trauma	Associated Injuries
MVA: Rotational force from spinning car	Combination of frontal and side impact–induced injuries
MVA: Rollover of vehicle	Multitude of external and internal injuries
MVA: Ejection from vehicle	Injuries at point of impact
MVA: Restrained driver or passenger	Compression of soft tissue organs, c-spine injuries, rib and sternal fractures, cardiac contusions, ruptured diaphragm
	Lap belt only: head, neck, facial, and chest injuries
	Shoulder strap only: severe neck injury, decapitation
	Air bag deployed: facial injuries, abrasions/burns of arms
Fall	
• Landing on feet	Compression fractures of lumbosacral spine
	Fractures of calcaneus
• Landing on buttocks	Compression fracture of lumbar vertebrae
	Pelvic fracture
	Coccyx fracture
Diving	Forceful cervical spine compression resulting in fracture, dislocation, and/or displacement of vertebral bone fragments into spinal canal
• Head first	
Blunt head trauma	Coup/contra-coup injury
• Person's moving head strikes a stationary object	Depressed skull fracture
	Cerebral hematoma, contusions, or laceration
Blunt chest trauma	Pulmonary contusion
• Moving object strikes a person's chest	Hemothorax
	Rib fractures
Crush injury to chest	Traumatic asphyxia
	• Crushing trauma to chest forces blood from heart via the superior vena cava to veins of the head, neck, and upper chest, causing subconjunctival and/or retinal hemorrhage, conjunctival edema, and characteristic deep violet skin color

Mechanisms of Injury: School Age and Adolescent (7 to 17 Years)

Common Mechanisms of Injury
Motor vehicle-related injuries
  Occupant
  Pedestrian
Bicycle-related injuries
Burns
  Flames
  Explosions
Suicide
  Ingestion
  Gunshot wounds
  Hanging
Minor trauma
  Superficial lacerations
Drowning
Falls
Sports-related injuries
Farm injuries
Penetrating trauma
  Stabbing
  Gunshot wounds

(continued)

Trauma	Associated Injuries
Assaults	Head/chest/abdomen: closed or open injuries, fractures, c-spine injury
Bicycle-related injuries	Head: closed or open injuries Chest: pulmonary/cardiac contusion, pneumothorax, rib fractures
Burns (flames, explosions)	Surface trauma; risk of multiple trauma exists
Drowning	Respiratory: acute respiratory distress syndrome (ARDS)
Falls	Head: cerebral swelling, epidural/subdural hematoma, skull fracture, c-spine injury Chest: pulmonary/cardiac contusion, hemo/pneumothorax Abdomen and misc: same as for MVAs
Farm injuries	Crush injuries
Minor trauma (superficial lacerations)	Surface trauma: lacerations, contusions
Motor vehicle accident (occupant, pedestrian)	Head: cerebral swelling, epidural/subdural hematoma, skull fractures, c-spine injuries Chest: pulmonary/cardiac contusion, hemothorax or pneumothorax rib fractures Abdomen: liver: fracture, laceration; spleen: hematoma, laceration, rupture; kidney: hematoma, contusion, hematuria; pancreas: contusion Misc: surface trauma, bony fractures
Penetrating trauma (stabbing, gunshot wounds)	Head/chest/abdomen: variety of injuries to internal organs
Sports-related injuries	Head: c-spine injuries Chest: rib fractures, pulmonary/cardiac contusions Abdomen: same as MVA possibilities
Suicide (ingestion, gunshot wounds, hanging)	Head: c-spine injury from hanging Chest/abdomen: variety of injuries from penetrating trauma, falls, MVAs

Appendix M

Mechanisms of Injury: Toddler and Preschooler (1 to 6 Years)

Common Mechanisms of Injury
Motor vehicle-related injuries
  Occupant
  Pedestrian
  Bicycle
Burns
  Scald and flame
Drownings
Ingestions
Minor surface trauma
Child abuse
Firearms (preschoolers)
Falls
Sledding
Choking
Animal bites

(*continued*)

Injury Pattern	Risk Factors	Associated Injuries
Abdomen	Pliable pelvic girdle fails to protect internal organs Proportionately larger abdominal organs Ribs do not protect upper abdominal contents Organs are in close proximity to each other Portion of bowel adheres to spine	Laceration, fracture, hematoma to solid organs (liver, spleen, kidney): MVAs, falls, abuse Hematoma to hollow organs: (esophagus, stomach, intestines): MVAs
Chest	Short trachea Compliant chest wall Mobile mediastinal structures Major vessels lack valves and predispose traumatic asphyxia	Pulmonary/cardiac contusions: MVAs, falls, sledding Pneumothorax: MVAs, falls, abuse Traumatic asphyxia: MVAs
Head	Thin, pliable bony structures predispose diffuse cerebral injuries	Diffuse cerebral swelling: MVAs, falls Subdural hematoma: abuse, falls Skull fractures: MVAs, falls, abuse, sledding
Long bones	Salter Harris Fractures (prior to puberty) Periosteum is stronger and allows bone to bend, leading to greenstick fractures	Long bone fractures: falls, MVAs, abuse, sports

Mechanisms of Injury: Infant (Birth to 1 Year)

Common Mechanisms of Injury
Airway compromise
  Choking
  Strangulation
  Suffocation
  Foreign body ingestion
Child abuse
  Shaken baby syndrome
Falls
Burns (scalds or flame)
Drownings
Poisonings
Baby walkers
Motor vehicle–related injuries
  With or without the proper use/placement of
    car seats

(*continued*)

Injury Pattern	Risk Factors	Associated Injuries
Abdomen	Pliable pelvic girdle does not protect internal organs	Laceration, fracture, rupture of solid organs (liver, spleen, kidney): MVAs, abuse, falls
	Portion of bowel adheres to spine	Hematoma, perforation of hollow organs
	Organs easily crushed between bony structure and injury object	(esophagus, stomach, intestines): MVAs, physical abuse
Chest	Tongue large in relation to oral cavity	Respiratory arrest: airway compromise, foreign body ingestion, obstruction
	Narrow airway	
	Obligate nose breather	Pneumothorax: MVAs, falls, abuse
	Short trachea	Pulmonary/cardiac contusion: MVAs, falls
	Pliable rib cage	
	Mobile mediastinal structures	
	Absence of valves in superior and inferior vena cava	
Head	Head large in proportion to body	Skull fractures: abuse, falls
	Poor head control as a result of weak neck muscles	Subdural hematoma: abuse
	Pliable body structures and vessels predispose infant to diffuse head injury	Retinal hemorrhages: abuse, traumatic asphyxia
		Diffuse cerebral swelling: MVAs, abuse, falls
		High cervical fracture: MVAs

Drugs of Abuse

Drug Name/ Type	Street Name	Method Used	Physical Effects	Mental Effects
Alcohol (a CNS depressant)	Booze, hooch, juice, brew	Swallowed in liquid form	Blurs vision; slurs speech, alters coordination; causes heart and liver damage, addiction, gastric and esophageal ulcers, brain damage, blackouts, hypoglycemia, anemia, Wernicke-Korsakoff syndrome, oral cancer, fetal alcohol syndrome; death from overdose	Scrambles thought process, impairs judgment, causes memory loss, alters perception, causes delirium, apathy
Cocaine (a CNS stimulant)	Coke, c-dust, snow, toot, white lady, blow, rock(s), crack, flake, big "C," happy dust, Bernice, fluff, caine, coconut, icing, mojo, zip	Smoked/ free based, inhaled/ snorted, injected, swallowed in powder, pill, or rock form	Rapidly metabolized, producing a brief high of <30 minutes; chronic use can result in cocaine psychosis, a condition similar to paranoid schizophrenia, intense psychological dependence, dilated pupils, profuse sweating, runny nose, dry mouth, tachycardia, hypertension, insomnia, anorexia, indifference to pain, destruction of nasal septum, heart and lung damage; death from overdose	Euphoria, illusion of mental or physical power, extreme mood swings, restlessness, hallucinations, paranoia, psychosis, severe depression, anxiety, formication

(continued)

Drug Name/ Type	Street Name	Method Used	Physical Effects	Mental Effects
CNS depressants— Barbiturates: phenobarbital (Luminal), amobarbital (Amytal), secobarbital (Seconal), pentobarbital (Nembutal), sodium pentothal	Reds, barbs, yellow jackets, red devils, blue devils, yellow submarine, blues and reds, idiot pills, sleepers, stumblers, downers	IV injection, suppository, swallowed in pill form	Drowsiness, slurred speech, skeletal muscle relaxation, poor muscle control, incoordination, nausea, slowed reaction time, involuntary eye movements, hypotension, bradycardia, bradypnea, constricted pupils, clammy skin, loss of appetite, penetrates the placental wall (addiction is passed to the baby); withdrawal is prolonged and severe: symptoms range from temporary psychosis to cardiac arrest; cellulitis at injection site, chronic use results in extreme psychological and physical addiction; death from overdose	Confusion, impaired judgment, impaired performance, anxiety and tension followed by a sense of calm, mood swings, forgetfulness
CNS depressants— Nonbarbiturates: methaqualone, quaalude, soper	Downers, ludes, soapers, wallbangers, lemons, lovers, quack, 714s, 300s	Swallowed in pill form	Same as barbiturates; physically and psychologically addictive; withdrawal is *very* difficult; severe interaction with alcohol; death from overdose	Same as barbiturates
CNS depressants— Tranquilizers, benzodi- azepines (reduce tension and anxiety without sedating): diazepam (Valium),	Downers	Injection, swallowed in pill form	Decreased reflex action, vision changes, muscle relaxation, hypotension, bradycardia, slurred speech, drowsiness, blurred vision; prolonged use causes severe physical and psychological addiction	Alteration in spatial judgment and sense of time, sense of calm, impaired judgment, confusion, depression, hallucinations

(*continued*)

Drug Name/ Type	Street Name	Method Used	Physical Effects	Mental Effects
chlordiazepox-ide (Librium), lorazepam (Ativan), oxazepam (Serax), alprazolam (Xanax)				
Hallucinogens (drugs that alter percep-tions of reality) PCP	Angel dust, killer, black whack, supergrass, peace pill, sherms, superweed, DOA, CJ, goon dust, dust joint, live one, mad dog, T-buzz, wobble weed, zombie	Swallowed in pill form, sprayed on a cigarette and smoked	Drooling, nystagmus, restlessness, incoordi-nation, rigid muscles, tachycardia, hypertension, superhuman strength, dulled sensations to touch and pain, impaired speech; death is common, but from accidents, not from overdose; extremely dangerous drug, as it is a narcotic, stimulant, depressant, and hallu-cinogen; a "trip" is a cycle of stimulation, depression, hallucination, and then repeats itself, lasting 2 to 14 hours	Disorientation, amnesia, anxiety, depression, confusion, agitation, violent behavior, hostility, suicidal urges, extreme personality changes
LSD	Acid, blue heaven, instant zen, purple hearts, pure love, sugar cubes, tail lights	Swallowed in liquid form, dropped on sugar cube, sprayed on paper tablet	Nausea, tachycardia, tachypnea, hyperthermia, hypertension, dilated pupils, diaphoresis, palpitations, incoordi-nation; trips last 4 to 14 hours; heightens all five senses	Altered perception of reality, psychotic disturbances, paranoia, synesthesia, hallucina-tions, mood swings, terrifying flashbacks
Mescaline, psilocybin mushrooms	Mesc, moon, peyote, buttons	Swallowed in natural form	Same as LSD	Same as LSD
Inhalants: Gasoline, airplane glue,		Inhaled or sniffed using a paper or	Incoordination, impaired vision, neuropathy, muscle weakness, anemia, vertigo,	Memory and thought impairment, depression, aggression, hostility, paranoia, abusive

(*continued*)

Drug Name/ Type	Street Name	Method Used	Physical Effects	Mental Effects
paint thinner, dry cleaner fluid		plastic bag or rag	headache, weight loss, nausea, vomiting, sneezing, coughing, nosebleeds, slurred speech, tachycardia, fatigue, dilated pupils, chemical smell on breath; brain, liver, and bone marrow damage; death by anoxia	behavior, mood swings, withdrawal from family and friends, violent behavior
Nitrous oxide	Laughing gas, whippets, buzz bomb, nitro	Inhaled or sniffed by mask or balloons		
Amyl nitrite, butyl nitrite	Poppers snappers, pearls, aimies, bolt, climax, thrust	Inhaled or sniffed from gauze or ampules		
Marijuana/ hashish (a CNS depressant)	Joint, grass, hash, pot, "J," Maryjane, reefer, Colombian locoweed, love weed	Smoked, swallowed in solid form	Interference with psycho-logical maturation, psychological dependence	Sensory distortion, decrease in motivation, forgetfulness, confusion, anxiety, paranoia
Narcotics (natural or synthetic drugs that contain or resemble opium; CNS depressants)				
Dilaudid	Dillys, cowboys	Swallowed in pill or liquid form, injected	Drowsiness, lethargy, hypotension, bradycardia, muscle weakness; death from overdose	Forgetfulness, sedation, sense of peace
Percodan	Perks, pink spoons			
Demerol	Peth			
Methadone	Dollies, amidone, fizzies			

(continued)

Drug Name/ Type	Street Name	Method Used	Physical Effects	Mental Effects
Codeine	Schoolboy cody, threes, fours	Swallowed in pill or liquid form		
Morphine	Mojo, morphy, mud, dreamer, Miss Emma	Smoked, IV injection	Tolerance occurs quickly; addiction occurs in as little as 1 to 3 weeks; withdrawal is painful with intense cramps, cold sweats, delirium, pain, fever, headaches, and seizures lasting about 4 days	Produces an intense orgasmic rush followed by euphoria, peace, and a comforting warmth; confusion, forgetfulness, stupor
Heroin	Horse, junk, dope, blanco, black pearl, Bonita, smack			
Stimulants (cause CNS stimulation) Amphetamines: Benzadrine, Biphetamine	Hi speed Lip poppers Speckled birds	Pill form, injected, snorted	Body enters a state of stress, anorexia, tachycardia, palpitations hypertension, inability to sleep, nasal and bronchial passages enlarge, restricted cerebral blood flow, dilated pupils, sweating, restlessness, muscle tremors, rapid and garbled speech, excessive activity, brain damage, seizures, CVA, coma; death from overdose; drug effects last 4 to 14 hours; "speeding" occurs with injection, causing user to go about 5 days without sleep; causes birth defects, extreme physical and psychological addiction	Extreme exhilaration and stimulation, inflated confidence, irritability, volatile and aggressive behavior, nervousness, mood swings, hallucinations, paranoia, formication, psychosis, hypomania
Dextroamphetamines: Dexedrine, Synatan, Appetral	Dexies, brownies, brown and clears			
Methamphetamines: Methedrine, Desoxyn, Ambar	Speed, meth, crystal, crank, crypto, ice, yellow bam			
Herbal stimulants (ephedra)	Ultimate Xphoria, herbal ecstasy, legal weed, buzz	Pill, powder, liquid	Same as above; often marketed as safe and legal alternatives to street drugs; increased sexual sensation, higher energy level,	Extreme exhilaration and stimulation, inflated confidence, reduced inhibitions, euphoria, happiness and

(*continued*)

Drug Name/ Type	Street Name	Method Used	Physical Effects	Mental Effects
	tablets, cloud 9, black lemonade, brainalizer, fungalore, herbal XTC, planet X, the drink, X tablets, brain wash, buzz tablets, fukola cola, love potion #69, naturally high, rave energy, love drug, Adam, XTC, X		tachycardia, sweating, body tremors, dilated pupils, muscle spasms, grinding of teeth, elevated blood pressure; easily obtainable over the Internet, through magazines, and at stores such as convenient markets, health food stores, and "head shops"	friendliness, empathy toward others, irritability, volatile and aggressive behavior, nervousness, mood swings, hallucinations, paranoia, formication, psychosis, hypomania
Anesthetics: GHB and analogs	Liquid X, liquid ecstasy, water, "G," easy lay	Oral	Onset is 10 to 20 minutes, duration is 2 to 3 hours; slow slurred speech, loss of muscle coordination, nausea, vomiting, bradycardia or tachycardia, hypotension, hypothermia; overdose: cardiac and respiratory arrest, seizures, incontinences of stool and urine, unconsciousness	Mood swings, amnesia, sleepiness, drunken appearance
Ketamine	K, super K, special K, God, jet, honey oil, blast, gas	Injected, snorted, smoked, oral, rectal	Onset is immediate if smoked or Injected; duration is 1 to 2 hours; about one-quarter the strength of PCP, depending on the dose used; sweating, slurred or slow speech, muscle rigidity, blank stare, elevated body temperature, tachycardia, loss of muscle coordination, hypertension, excess strength	Euphoria, paranoia, anxiety, disorientation, violence, agitation, insomnia, delusions, pain relief, intoxication, hallucinations, sleepy appearance, confusion

Poisonings

Substance and Common/Street Name	Clinical Signs and Symptoms
Acetaminophen (Tylenol)	Nausea, vomiting, anorexia, malaise, oliguria, increased liver enzymes Diffuse abdominal pain that becomes right upper quadrant abdominal pain
Alcohol	Sedation, relaxation, euphoria, memory loss, poor judgment, ataxia, slurred speech, nausea, vomiting, obtundation, coma In children, hypoglycemia occurs
Amphetamines (prescription: Ritalin, Tenuate, Preludin, Dexadrine; street: ice, crank, cat, jeff, ecstasy, mulka, crystal, speed)	CNS: agitation, delirium, hyperactivity, tremors, dizziness, mydriasis, CVA, headache, hyperreflexia, seizures, coma Psychiatric: euphoria, aggressive behavior, anxiety, hallucinations, compulsive repetitious actions Cardiopulmonary: palpitations, hypertensive crisis, tachycardia, reflex bradycardia, dysrhythmias, myocardial infarction, aortic dissection, pulmonary edema, respiratory distress
Anticholinergics (antihistamines, antiparkinsonian, cyclic antidepressants, antipsychotics, antispasmodics, mushrooms, Jimson weed)	Classic toxidrome: "mad as a hatter" (altered mental status); "hot as a hare" (hyperthermia); "red as a beet" (flushed skin); "dry as a bone" (dry skin and mucous membranes); "blind as a bat" (blurred vision secondary to mydriasis) (Rosen et al, 1999)
Arsenic	Acute ingestion: severe hemorrhagic gastroenteritis develops within hours, bone marrow depression, encephalopathy, cardiomyopathy, pulmonary edema, cardiac dysrhythmia, peripheral neuropathy Chronic ingestion: weakness, anorexia, hyperkeratosis, hyperpigmentation, hepatic injury, respiratory irritation, perforated nasal septum, tremor, peripheral neuropathy

(*continued*)

Substance and Common/Street Name	Clinical Signs and Symptoms
Barbiturates (Pentothal, Nembutal, Seconal, Mysoline, Phenobarbital)	CNS: lethargy, slurred speech, incoordination, ataxia, coma, hyporeflexia, nystagmus, stupor Cardiopulmonary: hypotension, bradycardia, respiratory depression, apnea Other: rhabdomyolysis, compartment syndrome, hypoglycemia
Benzodiazepines (Xanax, Librium, Clonopin, Valium, Dalmane, Ativan, Versed, Serax, Restoril, Halcion)	CNS: nystagmus, miosis, diplopia, impaired speech and coordination, amnesia, ataxia, confusion, somnolence, depressed deep tendon reflexes, dyskinesia Cardiopulmonary: hypotension, bradycardia, tachycardia (in response to the hypotension), respiratory depression, aspiration Other: hypothermia, rhabdomyolysis, skin necrosis
Beta-blockers (Atenolol, Brevibloc, Inderal, Lopressor, Tenormin, Timoptic)	CNS: seizures, coma, CNS depression Cardiopulmonary: hypotension, bradycardia, cardiac conduction delays, heart block, heart failure, bronchospasm, pulmonary edema, respiratory depression
Calcium-channel blockers (Cardizem, Procardia, Calan SR)	CNS: syncope, CNS depression, rare seizure, coma Cardiopulmonary: severe bradycardia, atrioventricular block, intraventricular conduction delays, ventricular dysrhythmias, congestive heart failure, respiratory depression, pulmonary edema Other: hyperglycemia, nausea, vomiting, ileus, hypotension, metabolic acidosis
Carbamazepine (oral antiseizure medications with a similar structure to tricyclic antidepressants)	CNS: ataxia, dizziness, drowsiness, nystagmus, hallucinations, combativeness, coma, seizures Cardiopulmonary: respiratory depression, aspiration pneumonia, hypotension, conduction disturbances, supraventricular tachycardia, bradycardia, EKG changes Other: urinary retention, hyponatremia, myoclonus
Carbon monoxide	CNS: headache, dizziness, ataxia, confusion, acute encephalopathy, syncope, seizures, coma Cardiopulmonary: chest pain, palpitations, dyspnea, myocardial infarction, tachycardia, hypotension Other: nausea, vomiting, decreased vision, retinal hemorrhage, lactic acidosis, rhabdomyolysis
Choral hydrate	CNS: headache, lightheadedness, ataxia, hyporeflexia, altered mental status Cardiopulmonary: hypotension, ventricular and supraventricular dysrhythmias, bradypnea Other: nausea, vomiting, abdominal pain, rash, pear-like breath odor
Cyanide	CNS: headache, confusion, syncope, seizures, coma, agitation, CNS stimulation Cardiopulmonary: tachycardia and hypertension progressing into bradycardia and hypotension
Digoxin	CNS: colored visual halos, blurred vision, agitation, lethargy, seizures, psychosis, hallucinations Cardiopulmonary: hypotension, cardiovascular collapse, bradycardia, Atria-ventricular block, paroxysmal atrial tachycardia, congestive heart failure

(continued)

Substance and Common/Street Name	Clinical Signs and Symptoms
Ethylene glycol	Other: nausea, vomiting, diarrhea, abdominal pain CNS: ataxia, slurred speech, irritability, cerebral edema, convulsions, coma Cardiopulmonary: tachycardia, bradycardia, hypotension, hypertension, pulmonary edema Other: nausea, vomiting, abdominal pain, hematemesis, acute renal failure, myalgia, hypocalcemia
Hallucinogens	CNS: restlessness, anxiety, incipient dread, distortions of reality, helplessness, coma, hyperreflexia Cardiopulmonary: tachycardia, hypertension, dysrhythmias, tachypnea, respiratory arrest Other: nausea, vomiting, hyperpyrexia, coagulopathies
Hydrocarbons	CNS: intoxication, headache, euphoria, slurred speech, lethargy, coma Cardiopulmonary: respiratory distress, cyanosis, aspiration, tachycardia, dysrhythmia Other: mucosal irritation, gastritis, diarrhea, acute renal failure
Hypoglycemic agents	CNS: headache, blurred vision, anxiety, irritability, confusion, stupor, coma, seizures Cardiopulmonary: respiratory distress, apnea, palpitations, tachycardia, hypertension, premature ventricular contractions Other: nausea, facial flushing, hypoglycemia, facial flushing, pallor
Iron	CNS: lethargy, seizures, coma Cardiopulmonary: tachycardia, tachypnea, hypotension Other: vomiting, abdominal pain, GI bleeding, diarrhea, renal failure, hepatic necrosis
Isoniazid	CNS: ataxia, hyperreflexia, agitation, hallucinations, psychosis, coma, seizures Cardiopulmonary: hypotension, tachycardia, shock, respiratory depression, Kussmaul respirations Other: hyperthermia, nausea, vomiting, severe anion gap, rhabdomyolysis
Lead (adult)	CNS: headache, confusion, altered mental status, seizures, nerve entrapment, motor neuropathy Cardiopulmonary/reproductive: hypertension, alterations in sperm count and quality Other: anorexia, dyspepsia, constipation, renal failure
Lead (pediatric)	CNS: cognitive dysfunction, decreased IQ, encephalopathy, irritability, headache, coma Hematologic: anemia, basophilic stippling Other: nausea, vomiting, abdominal pain, mild hearing loss
Lithium	CNS: lethargy, confusion, tremor, ataxia, slurred speech, hyperreflexia, clonus, dystonia Cardiopulmonary: EKG changes, respiratory failure Other: nausea, vomiting, diarrhea, diabetes insipidus, leukocytosis

(*continued*)

Substance and Common/Street Name	Clinical Signs and Symptoms
Methanol	CNS: inebriation, ataxia, seizures, coma, blurred vision, dilated pupils, headache, confusion Cardiopulmonary: hyperpnea, hypotension Other: metabolic acidosis, nausea, vomiting, abdominal pain
Nonsteroidal anti-inflammatories	CNS: drowsiness, dizziness, lethargy, seizures Cardiopulmonary: hypotension, tachycardia, hyperventilation, apnea Other: nausea, vomiting, abdominal pain, acute renal failure, metabolic acidosis
Organophosphates	CNS: headache, dizziness, tremors, anxiety, weakness, incoordination, convulsions, coma Cardiopulmonary: hypotension, bradycardia, atrioventricular block, asystole, bronchospasm, pulmonary edema Other: miosis, anorexia, abdominal cramps, salivation, lacrimation
Phencyclidines	CNS: impaired judgment, agitation, violent behavior, psychosis, paranoia, coma, seizures, dyskinesia Cardiopulmonary: hypertension, tachycardia, apnea Other: hyperthermia, acute renal failure, hypoglycemia
Phenothiazines	CNS: agitation, seizures, coma, extrapyramidal signs, tardive dyskinesia Cardiopulmonary: respiratory depression, pulmonary edema, tachycardia, EKG changes, V tach Other: hyperthermia, priapism, acute renal failure, constipation, ileus, agranulocytosis, anemia
Phenytoins	CNS: ataxia, nystagmus, cortical depression, confusion, slurred speech, coma, seizures Cardiopulmonary: hypotension, bradycardia, myocardial depression with rapid IV infusion Other: nausea, vomiting
Salicylates	CNS: tinnitus, deafness, delirium, seizures, coma, agitation, lethargy, confusion, cerebral edema Cardiopulmonary: hypotension, shock, tachypnea, noncardiac pulmonary edema, hyperventilation Other: nausea, vomiting, hepatic injury, acute renal insufficiency, hematemesis
Sympathomimetics	CNS: anxiety, headache, agitation, altered mentation, diaphoresis, stroke, seizures Cardiopulmonary: palpitations, chest pain, myocardial ischemia, tachydysrhythmias, hypertension Other: dilated pupils, dry mucous membranes, urinary retention, hyperthermia
Theophylline	CNS: tremor, agitation, nervousness, seizures Cardiopulmonary: hypotension, tachycardia, tachypnea, hypertension, dysrhythmias Other: nausea, vomiting, abdominal pain, hypokalemia, hyperglycemia, leukocytosis

(continued)

Substance and Common/Street Name	Clinical Signs and Symptoms
Toluene	CNS: depression, euphoria, ataxia, seizures, insomnia, headache, coma
	Cardiopulmonary: sudden cardiac death, dilated cardiomyopathy, myocardial infarction
	Other: renal failure, rhabdomyolysis, hematemesis, abdominal pain
Tricyclic antidepressants	CNS: agitation, tremors, seizures, drowsiness, lethargy, coma, ataxia, mania, dilated pupils
	Cardiopulmonary: hypotension, tachycardia, bradycardia, EKG changes, dysrhythmias
	Other: urinary retention, priapism, leukopenia, nausea, vomiting

Sources: Rosen et al., 1999; Dart, 2000.

Appendix Q

Biological Agents/Chemical Agents

Biological Agents						
Agent and Incubation Period	Signs, Symptoms, Sequelae, and Mode of Acquisition	Source	Vaccine Available	Contagious Between Humans	Treatment	Comments
Anthrax (inhaled): *Bacillus anthracis*; 7 days post-exposure	Resemble a common cold (fever, cough, malaise) that progress to severe dyspnea, diaphoresis, stridor, cyanosis, and shock Chest radiograph shows a mediastinal widening Gram-positive bacilli seen on blood smear and culture Hemorrhagic mediastinitis, thoracic lymphadenitis, and/or meningitis Inhalation of spores from contaminated animal products	Infected animal tissue Spores can live in the soil for years Biological warfare agent	Yes; approved for ages 18 to 65 3 injections given 2 weeks apart, followed by 3 more injections at 6, 12, and 18 months	Extremely unlikely	Early treatment is essential Penicillin Doxycycline Fluoroqui-nolones (Cipro) Special considera-tions for treatment of children, elderly, and pregnant women	90% to 100% of cases are fatal
Anthrax (cuta-neous): *Bacillus anthracis*; 7 days	Spores enter the skin Infection more likely with a cut or abrasion on the skin	Infected animal tissue, hair, fur, hides, leather	Yes; approved for ages 18 to 65	Rare, but can occur	Early treatment is essential Penicillin Doxycycline	Death rare if treated

(continued)

Biological Agents						
Agent and Incubation Period	Signs, Symptoms, Sequelae, and Mode of Acquisition	Source	Vaccine Available	Contagious Between Humans	Treatment	Comments
post-exposure	Infections begins with a raised, itchy bump that resembles a bug bite Within 1 to 2 days, a vesicle develops, followed by a painless ulcer 1 to 3 cm in diameter with a black necrotic center Lymph glands in the adjacent area may swell	Spores can live in the soil for years Biological warfare agent	3 injections given 2 weeks apart, followed by 3 more injections at 6, 12, and 18 months		Fluoroquinolones (Cipro) Special considerations for treatment of children, elderly, and pregnant women	20% of untreated cases are fatal
Anthrax (intestinal): *Bacillus anthracis*; 7 days post-exposure	Early symptoms: nausea, vomiting, malaise, anorexia, fever, acute inflammation of the GI tract Advanced symptoms: abdominal pain, vomiting blood, severe diarrhea Illness progresses rapidly Eating undercooked contaminated food	Infected animal tissue Spores can live in the soil for years Biological warfare agent	Yes; approved for ages 18 to 65 3 injections given 2 weeks apart, followed by 3 more injections at 6, 12, and 18 months	Extremely unlikely	Early treatment is essential Penicillin Doxycycline Fluoroquinolones (Cipro) Special considerations for treatment of children, elderly, and pregnant women	25% to 75% of cases are fatal
Botulism (food-borne): *Clostridium botulinum*; incubation depends on amount	Early symptoms: abdominal cramps, nausea, vomiting, diarrhea, and difficulty seeing, speaking, swallowing	Contaminated food from restaurants or home canned sources	Botulinum toxoid is available, but supplies are scarce and mass outbreaks	No	Antitoxin available from CDC; must be administered early in course of disease	Presents public health emergency Mortality rate = 8%

(*continued*)

Biological Agents						
Agent and Incubation Period	Signs, Symptoms, Sequelae, and Mode of Acquisition	Source	Vaccine Available	Contagious Between Humans	Treatment	Comments
and rate of toxin absorption: ranges from 2 hours to 8 days	Double or blurred vision, drooping eyelids, slurred speech, dry mouth Progresses to an acute, afebrile, symmetric, descending flaccid paralysis with multiple cranial nerve palsies, coma The most poisonous substance known; a major bioweapon threat due to its extreme potency, lethality, ease of production, transport, and misuse	Bacteria commonly found in the soil	of disease are rare		Supportive care	
Botulism (inhaled): Clostridium botulinum; incubation depends on amount and rate of toxin absorption, ranges from 12 to 80 hours	Ptosis, diplopia, blurred vision, dysarthria, dysphonia, dysphagia Progresses to an acute, afebrile, symmetric, descending flaccid paralysis with multiple cranial nerve palsies, coma The most poisonous substance known; a major bioweapon threat due to its extreme potency, lethality, ease of production, transport, and misuse	Man-made aerosolized form of the infection, created for use in bioterrorism	Botulinum toxoid is available, but supplies are scarce and mass outbreaks of disease are rare	No	Supportive care	Same as for food-borne botulism

(continued)

Biological Agents

Agent and Incubation Period	Signs, Symptoms, Sequelae, and Mode of Acquisition	Source	Vaccine Available	Contagious Between Humans	Treatment	Comments
Botulism (wound): *Clostridium botulinum*; incubation depends on amount and rate of toxin absorption	Double or blurred vision, drooping eyelids, slurred speech, dry mouth Progresses to an acute, afebrile, symmetric, descending flaccid paralysis with multiple cranial nerve palsies, coma Will NOT penetrate intact skin	Bacteria found in soil In recent years, black tar heroin from California is a prime source	As for food-borne and inhaled botulism	No	Antitoxin available from CDC; must be administered early in course of disease Supportive care	Infectious disease that would **NOT** result from bioterrorism
Botulism (intestinal): *Clostridium botulinum*	Lethargy, poor feeding, constipation, weakness, crying, and poor muscle tone Occasionally, susceptible patients may harbor *C. botulinum* in their intestinal tract (most often occurs in infants)	Bacteria commonly found in the soil	As for food-borne and inhaled botulism	No	Supportive care Antitoxin is not routinely given for infant botulism	Infectious disease that would **NOT** result from bioterrorism
Brucellosis (food-borne): *Brucella* species; incubation is variable	Flulike symptoms, such as fever, sweats, headache, back pain, and physical weakness. In severe cases, the patient may develop hepatitis, arthritis, spondylitis, anemia, leukopenia, thrombocytopenia, meningitis, uveitis, optic neuritis,	Ingestion of contaminated milk, dairy, or animal products High risk in unpasteurized milk, ice cream and cheeses	None available for humans	Extremely rare, although may possibly be transmitted through breast milk, sexual contact, or	Doxycycline and rifampin used in combination for 6 weeks Recovery takes a few weeks to several months	Mortality <2%

(continued)

Biological Agents						
Agent and Incubation Period	Signs, Symptoms, Sequelae, and Mode of Acquisition	Source	Vaccine Available	Contagious Between Humans	Treatment	Comments
Brucellosis (food-borne) (*cont'd*)	papilledema, and endocarditis Chronic symptoms may include recurrent fevers, joint pain, and fatigue			tissue transplantation		
Brucellosis (inhaled): *Brucella* species	Same as for food-borne brucellosis	Inhalation of aerosolized *Brucella*	None available for humans	See previous	See previous	See previous
Brucellosis (wound): *Brucella* species	Same as for food-borne brucellosis	Transmitted via skin abrasions while handling infected animals	None available for humans	See previous	See previous	See previous
Pneumonic plague: *Yersinia pestis*; incubation is 1 to 6 days post-exposure	Early signs are fever, headache, weakness, dyspnea, and productive cough (bloody or watery sputum) May see nausea, vomiting, abdominal pain, or diarrhea Acutely swollen and painful lymph nodes appear on the second day of infection, and the overlying skin is erythematous Pneumonia progresses over 2 to 4 days followed	Bacteria carried by rodents and their fleas Bioweapon usage would occur after aerosolization of the bacteria	None at this time; however, research is underway	Occurs through respiratory droplets during face-to-face contact	Early treatment is important Streptomycin Tetracycline Chloramphenicol Doxycycline Special considerations for treatment of children, elderly, and pregnant women Respiratory isolation	Death can occur in as little as 2 to 4 days

(*continued*)

Biological Agents						
Agent and Incubation Period	Signs, Symptoms, Sequelae, and Mode of Acquisition	Source	Vaccine Available	Contagious Between Humans	Treatment	Comments
	by septic shock and death				precautions, prophylactic antibiotic for close contacts of patient	
Smallpox: *Variola* virus; incubation is 7 to 17 days post-exposure	Initial symptoms are high fever, fatigue, headaches, and back aches Two to 3 days later, a rash appears in the mouth and on the face, arms, and legs, beginning as flat red lesions that evolve at the same rate; after a day or two the lesions become pus-filled and begin to crust early in the second week; scabs fall off after 3 to 4 weeks Patients with smallpox are most infectious during the first week of illness, although they are contagious until all skin scabs are healed In people exposed to smallpox, the vaccine can be	Infected saliva droplets	The United States has an emergency supply available (has not been routinely used since 1972)	Occurs through respiratory droplets during face-to-face contact Can also be transmitted by contaminated clothing or bedding	No proven treatment, although research for antivirals continues Supportive care should include intravenous fluids, antipyretics, and antibiotics for secondary infections Patients admitted to the hospital should be placed in negative-pressure rooms; staff should use standard precautions	Mortality rate = 30%

(*continued*)

Biological Agents						
Agent and Incubation Period	Signs, Symptoms, Sequelae, and Mode of Acquisition	Source	Vaccine Available	Contagious Between Humans	Treatment	Comments
Smallpox (*cont'd*)	given within 4 days to lessen or prevent the illness				to protect against spread of the disease	
Tularemia: *Francisella tularensis*; incubation is 1 to 14 days post-exposure	Initial symptoms are fever, pharyngitis, headache, body aches, and upper respiratory illness, rapidly progressing to bronchitis, pneumonia, pleuropneumonitis, bacteremia; may see nausea, weight loss, malaise with continued illness Inhalation would have the greatest adverse public health consequences; release in a densely populated area would result in an abrupt onset of a sick population (but slower progression than anthrax or plague) This is a dangerous bioweapon due to its extreme infectivity, ease of dissemination, and substantial capacity to cause illness and death	Contaminated arthropods, soil, animals, water, and vegetation Humans become infected by direct contact, ingestion, or inhaled infective aerosols	Vaccine available; not fully approved for general use	No	Individual treatment drugs of choice: streptomycin, gentamycin Mass casualty treatment drugs of choice: doxycycline, ciprofloxin Special considerations for children, pregnant women, and those with immunosuppression	<2% mortality rate

(*continued*)

Biological Agents					
Agent and Incubation Period	**Signs, Symptoms, Sequelae, and Mode of Acquisition**	**Source**	**Vaccine Available**	**Contagious Between Humans**	**Treatment**	**Comments**
Viral hemorrhagic fevers (VHF)	VHF is a term used to describe a severe multisystem syndrome in which the overall vascular system is damaged Initially, fever, fatigue, dizziness, muscle aches, weakness, and extreme fatigue are seen Severe infections will produce bleeding under the skin (petechiae), internal bleeding, or bleeding from body orifices; these patients will progress to shock, nervous system malfunction, coma, delirium, seizures, and/or renal failure VHF refers to a group of illnesses caused by several families of viruses: Arenaviruses (Argentine, Bolivian, Lassa); Bunyaviruses (Rift Valley, Hantavirus); Filoviruses (Ebola, Marburg); Flaviviruses (tick-borne, Kyasanur Forest)	Most VHFs are insect or animal borne The vectors for Ebola and Marburg viruses are un-known Humans become infected through contact with rodent's bodily fluids or when bitten by an arthro-pod	Available only for yellow fever and Argentine hemor-rhagic fever at this time No vaccines exist for the other VHFs	Humans may trans-mit some of these VHFs to other humans	There are no treatments for most of the VHFs Supportive care is given	Mortality rate varies with each VHF; most are between 50% and 90% mortality rate

(*continued*)

Biological Agents

Agent and Incubation Period	Signs, Symptoms, Sequelae, and Mode of Acquisition	Source	Vaccine Available	Contagious Between Humans	Treatment	Comments
Q fever: *Coxiella burnetii*; **incubation is 2 to 3 weeks post-exposure**	Sudden onset of high fevers (104°F to 105°F), severe headache, malaise, myalgia, confusion, sore throat, chills, sweats, nonproductive cough, nausea, vomiting, diarrhea, abdominal pain, chest pain Fever lasts for 1 to 2 weeks Thirty percent to 50% of patients develop pneumonia This agent is highly infectious and resistant to heat, drying, and most disinfectants; it easily becomes airborne and is inhaled by humans and therefore is at risk of abuse by bioterrorists Chronic Q fever occurs when infection persists for >6 months; these patients are prone to endocarditis	Infected milk, urine, feces, amniotic fluid of animals Humans are infected by inhaling dried, contaminated particles Ingestion of contaminated milk may produce illness	Yes, although not commercially available in the United States	Rare	Q fever: doxycycline; most efficient when started within first 3 days of illness Chronic Q fever: doxycycline with quinolones for at least 4 years or doxycycline with hydrochloroquine for 1.5 to 3 years	Q fever: <2% mortality rate Chronic Q fever: 65% mortality rate

Sources: Arnon, 2001; CDC, 2001; Inglesby, 2000; CDC, 1997; Henderson, 1999; Dennis, 2001. Reprinted with permission from www.rnceus.com.

(*continued*)

Chemical Agents

Agents and Descriptions	Onset of Symptoms Post-Exposure	Signs and Symptoms, Routes of Exposure	Action, Risks	Decontamination and Treatment
Nerve agents				
Sarin; Pure liquid is clear, colorless, tasteless; becomes brown with aging	Immediately if inhaled; may be several hours if it touches the skin	Runny nose, watery eyes, drooling, blurred vision, headache, excessive sweating, chest tightness, difficulty breathing, nausea, vomiting, loss of bowel/bladder control, muscle cramps, twitching, confusion, convulsions, paralysis, and coma — Can enter the body by inhalation, ingestion, through the eyes and skin	Chemicals that attack the nervous system by binding w/ acetylcholinesterase, allowing acetylcholine to overstimulate the glands and voluntary muscles until they fail. Lethal; 1 drop on the skin can cause death in less than 15 minutes	**Skin**: Remove contaminated clothing (double bag in plastic bags and seal) and wash skin with large amount of soap and water or 5% bleach. Rinse well with water. **Eyes**: Immediately flush eyes with water for 10 to 15 minutes; do NOT cover eyes with patches afterward. **Ingestion**: Do NOT induce vomiting. If patient alert and able to swallow, immediately administer activated charcoal. **Vapor**: Remove outer clothing and place in sealed double bag. Care for exposed skin as above. **Emergency treatment and antidotes**: Maintain airway, cardiac monitor, IVs, monitor vital signs. Follow ACLS protocols. Administer atropine (2 mg for adults, 0.05 to 0.1 mg/kg for children) every 5 to 10 minutes until respiratory status stabilizes; antidote (2-PAM CL); diazepam for seizures (barbiturates and phenytoin are not effective)
VX; amber colored, tasteless, and odorless oily liquid	Onset of symptoms varies based on route of exposure VX absorbs very rapidly	Runny nose, watery eyes, drooling, excessive sweating, chest tightness, dyspnea, pinpoint pupils, nausea, vomiting,	Kills by binding acetylcholinesterase; this causes constant stimulation of glands and voluntary	**Skin**: Remove contaminated clothes and wash skin with large amounts of soap and water, 10% sodium carbonate, or 5% liquid household bleach. Rinse well with water. Administer antidote only if local sweating and muscular twitching are present.

(continued)

Chemical Agents				
Agents and Descriptions	Onset of Symptoms Post-Exposure	Signs and Symptoms, Routes of Exposure	Action, Risks	Decontamination and Treatment
VX (*cont'd*)	through the eyes At least 100 times more toxic than Sarin when entering through the skin and twice as toxic by inhalation	abdominal cramps, in-continence of bowel or bladder, twitching, headache, confusion, coma, or seizures Can enter the body by inhalation, ingestion, through the eyes and skin Death can occur within 15 min-utes of absorp-tion of fatal dosage.	muscles until ultimate fatigue and a cessation of breathing ability Extremely lethal and persis-tent; can last for months in cold weather; evaporates 1,500 times slower than water	**Eyes:** *Immediately* flush eyes with water for 10 to 15 minutes, then place respiratory protective mask. Use antidote only if more symptoms than just miosis occur. VX absorbs 100 times faster through the eyes than Sarin does. **Ingestion:** Do NOT induce vom-iting. **Inhalation:** Use positive-pressure, full-face breathing mask. Do NOT perform mouth-to-mouth on a patient with VX exposure! Immediately administer nerve agent antidote. **Emergency treatment and antidotes:** Maintain airway, cardiac monitor, IVs, monitor vital signs. Follow ACLS protocols. Administer atropine (2 mg for adults, 0.05 to 0.1 mg/kg for children) every 5 to 10 minutes until respiratory status stabilizes; antidote (2-PAM CL); diazepam for seizures (barbiturates and phenytoin are not effective)
GF (cyclohexyl sarin); colorless and odorless liquid in pure form	Depending on the dose, onset of symptoms within minutes or hours Rapid absorp-tion through the eyes	Runny nose, miosis, headache, dyspnea, chest tightness, cough, drool-ing, excessive sweating, copious sinus secretions, nausea,	Organophos-phorus compound, a lethal cholinesterase inhibitor similar in action to sarin	**Skin:** Remove contaminated clothes and wash skin with large amounts of soap and water, 10% sodium carbonate, or 5% liquid household bleach. Rinse well with water. Administer antidote only if local sweating and muscular twitching is present. **Eyes:** *Immediately* flush eyes with water for 10 to 15 minutes,

(continued)

Chemical Agents

Agents and Descriptions	Onset of Symptoms Post-Exposure	Signs and Symptoms, Routes of Exposure	Action, Risks	Decontamination and Treatment
		vomiting, abdominal cramps, diarrhea, incontinence of bowel and bladder, muscle twitching and weakness, confusion, apnea, coma, death Can enter the body by inhalation, ingestion, through the eyes and skin		then place respiratory protective mask. Use antidote only if more symptoms than just miosis occur. **Ingestion**: Do NOT induce vomiting. Immediately administer nerve agent antidote. **Inhalation**: Use positive-pressure, full face, self-contained breathing apparatus. For severe signs, immediately administer nerve agent antidote and oxygen. Do NOT perform mouth-to-mouth resuscitation if face is contaminated with GF. **Emergency treatment and antidotes**: Maintain airway, cardiac monitor, IVs, monitor vital signs. Follow ACLS protocols. Administer atropine (2 mg for adults, 0.05 to 0.1 mg/kg for children) every 5 to 10 minutes until respiratory status stabilizes; antidote (2-PAM CL); diazepam for seizures (barbiturates and phenytoin are not effective)

Pulmonary agents

Agents and Descriptions	Onset of Symptoms Post-Exposure	Signs and Symptoms, Routes of Exposure	Action, Risks	Decontamination and Treatment
Nitrogen oxide; red/brown gas or a yellow liquid with pungent odor	The substance and vapor irritate the eyes, skin, and respiratory tract. Effects may be delayed	Cough, wheezing, sore throat, dizziness, headache, sweating, dyspnea, vomiting, or redness at point of contact (eyes, skin)	Causes lung edema Exposure of high amounts can cause death	**Skin**: Rinse with plenty of water then remove contaminated clothing and rinse again. Refer for medical attention. **Eyes**: Flush eyes with water for 10 to 15 minutes (be sure to remove contact lenses), then refer for medical attention. **Ingestion**: Rinse mouth with copious amounts of water.

(continued)

Chemical Agents				
Agents and Descriptions	Onset of Symptoms Post-Exposure	Signs and Symptoms, Routes of Exposure	Action, Risks	Decontamination and Treatment
Nitrogen oxide (*cont'd*)		Can enter the body by inhalation or ingestion		**Inhalation:** Apply oxygen, place in sitting position. Seek medical evaluation.
Chlorine; green/ yellow gas with pungent odor	Effects may be delayed	Very corrosive effects Tearing of the eyes, headache, sore throat, cough, dyspnea, burning sensation, lung edema, frostbite, burns to the skin, nausea, eye pain, blurred vision Enters the body by inhalation	Corrosive effects to lungs, skin, and eyes Chronic exposure results in erosion of the teeth, chronic bronchitis Overexposure can cause death	**Skin:** Remove contaminated clothing, then rinse skin with plenty of water or a shower. Seek medical help for burns. **Eyes:** Flush eyes with water for 10 to 15 minutes (be sure to remove contact lenses), then refer for medical attention. **Inhalation:** Apply oxygen, place in sitting position. May need artificial ventilation. Seek medical evaluation.
Sulfur dioxide; colorless gas or compressed liquefied gas with pungent odor	Inhalation symptoms may be delayed Contact with skin can cause immediate frostbite	Frostbite to the skin, eye pain with redness and severe burns, sore throat, cough, dyspnea, lung edema, reflex spasm of the larynx, respiratory arrest, death Enters the body by inhalation	Strong irritant to the eyes and respiratory tract Repeated or prolonged exposure can cause asthma	**Skin:** Remove contaminated clothing, then rinse with plenty of water. Do NOT remove clean clothing. Seek medical help for frostbite. **Eyes:** Flush eyes with water for 10 to 15 minutes (be sure to remove contact lenses), then refer for medical attention. **Inhalation:** Apply oxygen, place in sitting position. May need artificial ventilation. Seek medical evaluation.
Phosgene; colorless gas, colorless to yellow	Inhalation symptoms may be delayed	Frostbite to the skin, eye pain with redness and severe burns, blurred	Corrosive to skin, respiratory tract, and eyes	**Skin:** Remove contaminated clothing, then rinse with plenty of water. Do NOT remove clean clothing. Seek medical help for frostbite.

(*continued*)

Chemical Agents

Agents and Descriptions	Onset of Symptoms Post-Exposure	Signs and Symptoms, Routes of Exposure	Action, Risks	Decontamination and Treatment
compressed liquefied gas with characteris tic odor	Contact with skin can cause immediate frostbite	vision, sore throat, cough, dyspnea, lung edema, death Enters the body by inhalation	Long-term exposure may result in lung fibrosis	**Eyes:** Flush eyes with water for 10 to 15 minutes (be sure to remove contact lenses), then refer for medical attention. **Inhalation:** Apply oxygen, place in sitting position. May need artificial ventilation. Seek medical evaluation.
Titanium tetra-chloride; colorless to light yellow liquid with pungent odor	Symptoms may be delayed	Red painful eyes with burns, skin blisters, cough, dysp-nea, chest tightness, abdominal pain, shock, coma Enters the body by inhalation or ingestion	Corrosive to skin, eyes, respiratory, and GI tract; can cause permanent eye damage Long-term exposure may result in lung impairment	**Skin:** Remove contaminated clothing, rinse with plenty of water, then wash with soap and water **Eyes:** Flush eyes with water for 10 to 15 minutes (be sure to remove contact lenses), then refer for medical attention. **Ingestion:** Rinse mouth. Do NOT induce vomiting. Seek medical attention immediately **Inhalation:** Apply oxygen, place in sitting position. May need artificial ventilation. Seek medical evaluation.
Blister agents				
Lewisite; amber to dark brown liquid with a strong, penetrating geranium odor; the pure compound is a colorless, odorless, oily liquid	Immediate symptoms with eye exposure, inhalation, or ingestion Skin contact produces symptoms within 30 minutes	Eyelid swelling, severe eye pain, iritis, copious sinus drainage, violent sneez-ing, cough, frothing mucus, lung edema, large skin blisters and burns, diarrhea, hypothermia, hypotension	Causes blind-ness within 1 minute of exposure Nonfatal hemolysis results in anemia Metabolites excreted by liver cause focal necrosis of liver, bil-iary passages, and intestine	**Skin:** Immediately wash skin and clothes with 5% sodium hypochlorite or household bleach within 1 minute of exposure, then cut and remove contaminated cloth. Rewash skin again with 5% liquid household bleach. Then wash contaminated skin a third time with soap and water. **Eyes:** Immediately flush eyes with water for 10 to 15 minutes. **Ingestion:** Rinse mouth. Do NOT induce vomiting. Give patient milk to drink.

(continued)

Chemical Agents				
Agents and Descriptions	Onset of Symptoms Post-Exposure	Signs and Symptoms, Routes of Exposure	Action, Risks	Decontamination and Treatment
Lewisite (*cont'd*)		Severe irritation and lung edema; can cause systemic poisoning, hemoconcentration, shock, and death Can enter the body by inhalation, ingestion, through the eyes and skin	Long-term exposure can cause chronic lung impairment and cancer	**Inhalation:** Apply oxygen, place in sitting position. May need artificial ventilation. Do NOT perform mouth-to-mouth resuscitation if facial contamination has occurred.
Mustard gas; pure liquid is colorless and odorless; agent-grade material is yellow, brown, or black with a sweet-type odor of garlic or horseradish	Rapid penetration of moist mucous membranes and skin Delayed severe symptoms of the respiratory tract	Severe tearing and pain of eyes with possible blindness, sneezing, coughing, anorexia, diarrhea, fever, skin blisters Can enter the body by inhalation, ingestion, or through the eyes and skin; tender skin, mucous membranes, and perspiration-covered skin are more vulnerable	Causes delayed severe damage to the respiratory tract and cytotoxic action on hematopoietic tissues Lethal doses are carcinogens and teratogens Distilled mustard is nearly pure, while mustard gas is only 70% to 80% pure	**Skin:** Immediately wash skin and clothes with 5% sodium hypochlorite or household bleach within 1 minute of exposure, then cut and remove contaminated cloth. Flush skin again with 5% sodium hypochlorite solution, then wash contaminated skin a third time with soap and water. **Eyes:** Immediately flush eyes with water for 10 to 15 minutes. Do not cover with bandages. Use dark goggles or glasses. **Ingestion:** Do NOT induce vomiting. Give patient milk to drink. **Inhalation:** Apply oxygen, place in sitting position. May need artificial ventilation. Do NOT perform mouth-to-mouth resuscitation if facial contamination has occurred.

(*continued*)

Chemical Agents

Agents and Descriptions	Onset of Symptoms Post-Exposure	Signs and Symptoms, Routes of Exposure	Action, Risks	Decontamination and Treatment
Blood agents				
Arsine; colorless compressed liquefied gas with a characteristic odor	Immediate to delayed symptoms, depending on exposure	Causes immediate frostbite when contact made with eyes or skin Headache, confusion, dizziness, nausea, vomiting, abdominal pain, dyspnea, lung edema, kidney failure, damage to blood cells, death Enters the body by inhalation	Chronic exposure is carcinogenic to humans	**Skin:** Remove contaminated clothing, then rinse with plenty of water. Do NOT remove clean clothing. Seek medical help for frostbite. **Eyes:** Flush eyes with water for 10 to 15 minutes, follow with an immediate eye exam. **Inhalation:** Apply oxygen, place in sitting position. May need artificial ventilation.
Cyanogen chloride; colorless compressed liquefied gas with a pungent odor	Effects of exposure may be delayed	Causes immediate frostbite when contact made with eyes or skin Sore throat, severe tearing, confusion, drowsiness, unconsciousness, nausea, vomiting, lung edema Enters the body by inhalation or absorbed through the skin	Overexposure results in death	**Skin:** Remove contaminated clothing, then rinse with plenty of water. Do NOT remove clean clothing. Seek medical help for frostbite. **Eyes:** Flush eyes with water for 10 to 15 minutes, follow with an immediate eye exam. **Inhalation:** Apply oxygen, place in sitting position. May need artificial ventilation.

(continued)

Chemical Agents

Agents and Descriptions	Onset of Symptoms Post-Exposure	Signs and Symptoms, Routes of Exposure	Action, Risks	Decontamination and Treatment
Hydrogen chloride; colorless compressed liquefied gas with a pungent odor	Highly corrosive; symptoms may begin immediately or be delayed	Corrosive, deep, severe burns to eyes and skin Sore throat, blurred vision, coughing, dyspnea, lung edema, burning sensation Enters the body through inhalation	Long-term exposure may cause erosion to the teeth or chronic bronchitis	**Skin**: Remove contaminated clothing, then rinse with plenty of water. Seek treatment for burns. **Eyes**: Flush eyes with water for 10 to 15 minutes; follow with an immediate eye exam. **Inhalation**: Apply oxygen, place in sitting position. May need artificial ventilation.
Hydrogen cyanide; colorless gas or liquid with a characteristic odor	Highly irritating; symptoms may be immediate or delayed	Headache, confusion, drowsiness, dyspnea, loss of consciousness, nausea, skin and eye redness and pain, burning sensation Enters the body through inhalation, ingestion, eye and skin absorption Easily absorbed as a vapor or through the skin or eyes	May injure CNS, respiratory and circulatory systems Exposure may cause death	**Skin**: Flush skin with plenty of water or take a shower. Wear gloves when administering first aid. **Eyes**: Immediately flush eyes with water for 10 to 15 minutes then seek eye exam. **Ingestion**: Rinse mouth immediately. Do NOT induce vomiting. **Inhalation**: Apply oxygen, place in sitting position. May need artificial ventilation. Avoid mouth-to-mouth resuscitation.

Sources: CDC, 2001; CDC, 2002.

(*continued*)

Pre-Hospital Triage of Mass Casualty Patients: Nerve Agents

Triage Priority	Priority Description	Current State	Clinical Signs
Immediate	Patients who require lifesaving care within a short period of time Emergency care must be available and of short duration This care may include emergency measures that are performed within a few minutes' time, such as intubation or antidote administration	Unconscious Talking but unable to walk Moderate to severe effects on two or more organs or systems (e.g., respiratory, GI)	Seizing or postictal Severe respiratory distress Cardiac arrest (recovered)
Delayed	Patients with severe injuries in need of major surgery, require hospitalization, or other care, but a delay in care will not adversely affect the outcome of this patient, e.g., internal stabilization of a fracture	Recovering from recent exposure or antidote administration	Diminished secretions Improving or stable respiratory status
Minimal	Patients who have minor injuries who can be helped by nonmedical personnel and who will not require hospitalization	Walking and talking	Miosis Rhinorrhea Mild to moderate dyspnea
Expectant	Patients with severe, life-threatening conditions who probably would not survive even with the best of medical attention Patients with injuries that require attention from many medical personnel but low chance of survival does not justify the use of limited medical resources As this mass casualty event changes, these patients may be re-triaged once additional medical resources become available	Unconscious	Cardiac arrest Respiratory arrest

Sources: CDC, 2001; ATSDR, 2001.

(continued)

Pre-Hospital Antidote Management When Military Mark I Kits Are Not Available

Patient Age	Mild Symptoms (Localized Sweating, Difficulty Breathing, Nausea, Vomiting, Diarrhea, Muscle Fasciculations, Weakness)	Severe Symptoms (Apnea, Seizures, Flaccid Paralysis, Unconsciousness)
Infant: <2 years old	Atropine: 0.05 mg/kg IM 2-PAM Cl: 15 mg/kg IM	Atropine: 0.1 mg/kg IM 2-PAM Cl: 25 mg/kg IM
Child: 2–10 years old	Atropine: 1 mg IM 2-PAM Cl: 15 mg/kg IM	Atropine: 2 mg IM 2-PAM Cl: 25 mg/kg IM
Adolescent: >10 years old	Atropine: 2 mg IM 2-PAM Cl: 15 mg/kg IM	Atropine: 4 mg IM 2-PAM Cl: 25 mg/kg IM
Adult	Atropine: 2 to 4 mg IM 2-PAM Cl: 600 mg IM	Atropine: 6 mg IM 2-PAM Cl: 1800 mg IM
Frail elderly	Atropine: 1 mg IM 2-PAM Cl: 10 mg/kg IM	Atropine: 2 to 4 mg IM 2-PAM Cl: 25 mg/kg IM

Sources: CDC, 2001; ATSDR, 2001.

ALERTS

- 2-PAM Cl solution needs to be reconstituted from the vial containing 1 g of desiccated 2-PAM Cl with 3 mL of saline, 5% distilled water, or sterile water; shake well. Resulting solution is 3.3 mL of 300 mg/mL.
- Assisted ventilation should be started after the administration of the antidote for severe cases of exposure.
- Repeat the atropine every 5 to 10 minutes until secretions have diminished and breathing has returned to baseline.

(continued)

Emergency Department Antidote Management

Patient Age	Mild Symptoms (Localized Sweating, Difficulty Breathing, Nausea, Vomiting, Diarrhea, Muscle Fasciculations, Weakness)	Severe Symptoms (Apnea, Seizures, Flaccid Paralysis, Unconsciousness)
Infant: <2 years old	Atropine: 0.05 mg/kg IM or 0.02 mg/kg IV 2-PAM Cl: 15 mg/kg IV slowly	Atropine: 0.1 mg/kg IM or 0.02 mg/kg IV 2-PAM Cl: 15 mg/kg IV slowly
Child: 2–10 years old	Atropine: 1 mg IM 2-PAM Cl: 15 mg/kg IV slowly	Atropine: 2 mg IM 2-PAM Cl: 15 mg/kg IV slowly
Adolescent: >10 years old	Atropine: 2 mg IM 2-PAM Cl: 15 mg/kg IV slowly	Atropine: 4 mg IM 2-PAM Cl: 15 mg/kg IV slowly
Adult	Atropine: 2 to 4 mg IM 2-PAM Cl: 15 mg/kg (1 g) IV slowly	Atropine: 6 mg IM 2-PAM Cl: 15 mg/kg (1 g) IV slowly
Frail elderly	Atropine: 1 mg IM 2-PAM Cl: 5 to 10 mg/kg IV slowly	Atropine: 2 mg IM 2-PAM Cl: 5 to 10 mg/kg IV slowly

Sources: CDC, 2001; ATSDR, 2001.

ALERTS

- 2-Pam Cl solution may need to be reconstituted from the vial containing 1 gram of desiccated 2-PAM Cl with 3 mL of saline, 5% distilled water, or sterile water; shake well. Resulting solution is 3.3 mL of 300 mg/mL.
- Use phentolamine for hypertension induced by 2-PAM (5 mg IV for adults, 1 mg IV for children).
- Use diazepam for seizure control (0.2 to 0.5 mg IV for children <5 years old; 1 mg IV for children >5 years old; 5 mg IV for adults).
- Repeat atropine every 5 to 10 minutes until secretions have diminished & dyspnea relieved (for infants, use 2 mg IM or 1 mg IV)

Appendix R

Communicable Diseases, Colds Versus Flu, and Sexually Transmitted Diseases

Communicable Diseases			
Disease	Mode of Transmission	Incubation Period (Days)	Contagious Period (Days)
Acquired immunodeficiency syndrome (AIDS)/human immunodeficiency virus (HIV)	Blood, breast milk, body tissues, fluids exchanged during sexual contact Other body fluids: saliva, urine, tears, bronchial secretions (especially if blood is present)	Variable incubation rates Virus exposure to seroconversion (HIV+): about 1 to 3 months HIV+ to AIDS: from <1 year to 10 years	Although unknown, it is believed to begin just after onset of HIV and extend throughout life
Botulism	Contaminated food products	Within 12 to 36 hours of consumption, up to several days	Not contagious from secondary person-to-person contact
Bronchiolitis	Respiratory	4 to 6 days	Onset of cough until 7 days
Chancroid	Direct sexual contact with open or draining lesions	3 to 5 days, up to 14 days	Until treated with antibiotic and lesions healed—usually about 1 to 2 weeks
Chickenpox (varicella)	Direct person-to-person contact, respiratory droplets	Commonly 14 to 16 days	One to 5 days before the onset of the rash until all sores have crusted over—usually 10 to 21 days.
Chlamydia	Sexual intercourse	Approximately a minimum of 7 to 14 days	Unknown

(continued)

Communicable Diseases

Disease	Mode of Transmission	Incubation Period (Days)	Contagious Period (Days)
"Cold," cough, croup	Respiratory	2 to 5 days	Onset of runny nose and/or cough until fever is gone
Conjunctivitis Viral	Direct or indirect contact	1 to 12 days	4 to 14 days after onset of symptoms (minimally contagious)
Bacterial	Respiratory, direct contact with eye drainage	24 to 72 hours	Until treated with antibiotics
Fifth disease	Respiratory	Variable; 4 to 20 days	7 days before rash develops, probably not communicable after rash starts
Giardia	Fecal contamination of food or water	3 to 25 days	Entire period of infection, often months
Gonorrhea	Sexual contact	2 to 7 days	Continues until treatment begins
Hand, foot, and mouth disease (Coxsackie virus)	Direct contact with nasal or throat secretions, fecal material droplets	3 to 6 days	Onset of mouth ulcers until fever gone—perhaps as long as several weeks with fecal contamination
Hepatitis A	Fecal-oral route, food contamination	15 to 50 days	During last half of incubation period until after first week of jaundice
Hepatitis B	Blood, saliva, semen, vaginal fluid	45 to 180 days	Infective many weeks before onset of first symptom, until completion of acute clinical course of infection
Hepatitis C	Blood and plasma, percutaneous exposure	2 weeks to 6 months	From 1+ weeks before onset of Symptoms; may persist indefinitely
Herpes simplex Type 1	Saliva	2 to 12 days	From onset of sores to 7 weeks after recovery from stomatitis
Type 2	Sexual contact (oral or genital)	2 to 12 days	7 to 12 days

(*continued*)

Communicable Diseases			
Disease	Mode of Transmission	Incubation Period (Days)	Contagious Period (Days)
Herpes (varicella) zoster/shingles	Soiled dressings or articles	Can be 2 to 3 weeks	One to 5 days before the onset of the rash until all sores have crusted over—usually 10 to 21 days
Impetigo			
Staph	Hand-to-skin contact	4 to 10 days	Until draining lesions heal
Strep	Respiratory droplet, direct contact	1 to 3 days	Untreated: weeks or months; treated: 24 hours on antibiotics
Influenza	Airborne, direct contact	1 to 3 days	Children: 7 days; adults: 3 to 5 days
Kawasaki	Unknown, seasonal variation	Unknown	Unknown
Legionnaire pneumonia	Airborne	2 to 10 days	Person-to-person: none
Lice			
Head/body	Direct contact, indirect contact with objects	7 to 13 days	Continuous if alive, until first treatment; live off host for 7 to 21 days
Pubic (crabs)	Sexual contact	Egg-to-egg cycle lasts 3 weeks	Live off host for 2 days
Lyme disease	Tickborne	3 to 32 days	Person-to-person: none
Measles (rubeola)	Airborne, direct contact w/nasal secretions	7 to 18 days	Before the onset of symptoms to 4 days after the appearance of the rash
Meningitis			
Bacterial: Meningococcal	Direct contact, respiratory, droplet from nose and mouth	2 to 10 days	Usually after 24 hours on antibiotic therapy
Bacterial: Haemophilus	Droplet from nose and mouth	2 to 4 days	Noncommunicable within 24 to 48 hours on antibiotic therapy
Viral	Varies with specific infectious agent		Variable; often approximately 7 days
Mononucleosis	Saliva	4 to 6 weeks	Prolonged, possibly a year
Pertussis	Direct contact, airborne droplet	6 to 20 days	Gradually decreases over 3 weeks
Pinworms	Direct transfer (anus to mouth), indirect contact (infested bed, etc.)	2 to 6 weeks	As long as females are alive, eggs survive for about 2 weeks

(continued)

Communicable Diseases

Disease	Mode of Transmission	Incubation Period (Days)	Contagious Period (Days)
Rabies	Saliva, direct contact (bite, scratch), indirect contact	3 to 8 weeks	3 to 7 days before the onset of symptoms
Ringworm			
Tinea capitis (scalp)	Direct skin-to-skin, indirect contact (cloth seats, combs, etc.)	10 to 14 days	Viable fungus may persist on contaminated articles for long periods of time
Tinea corporis (body)	Direct or indirect contact with infected people, articles, floors, benches, animals, shower stalls	4 to 10 days	While lesions are present and as long as viable fungus remains on articles
Rocky Mountain spotted fever	Tickborne	3 to 14 days	Noncommunicable person-to-person; tick remains infective for life, as long as 18 months
Roseola	Unknown, possibly saliva	10 to 15 days	Onset of fever until rash is gone
Rotavirus	Fecal-oral route, possible respiratory	24 to 72 hours	Average 4 to 6 days
Rubella	Direct contact with nasal secretions, droplet	14 to 23 days	One week before to at least 4 days after onset of rash
Salmonella	Ingestion of contaminated food	6 to 72 hours	Throughout the course of infection
Scabies	Direct skin-to-skin contact	2 to 6 weeks	Until mites and eggs are destroyed
Scarlet fever	Large respiratory droplet, direct contact	1 to 3 days	Untreated: 10 to 21 days; treated: 24 hr of antibiotic therapy
Shigella	Fecal-oral route, ingestion of contaminated food	12 to 96 hours	During acute infection until infectious agent no longer in feces (about 4 weeks)
Sore throat			
Strep	Large respiratory droplet, direct contact	1 to 3 days	Untreated: 10 to 21 days; treated: after 24 hrs of antibiotic therapy

(continued)

Communicable Diseases

Disease	Mode of Transmission	Incubation Period (Days)	Contagious Period (Days)
Viral	Direct contact, inhalation of airborne droplet	1 to 5 days	Onset of sore throat until fever gone
Syphilis	Direct contact with moist lesions and body fluids	10 days to 3 months	Untreated: variable and indefinite; treated: after 24 to 48 hr of antibiotic therapy
Tetanus	Spores enter open wound	3 to 21 days	Noncommunicable from person-to-person
Trichomoniasis	Sexual contact through vaginal or urethral secretions	4 to 24 days	Untreated: may be symptom-free carrier for years
Tuberculosis	Airborne droplet	4 to 12 weeks	Degree of communicability depends on many factors; treated: within a few weeks; children usually not infectious

Source: Grossman, V. A. (2003). *Quick Reference to Triage* (2nd ed.). Philadelphia: Lippincott Williams & Wilkins.

"Cold" Versus Flu Symptom Comparison

Symptom	"Cold"	Flu
Fever	Rare	Usually high (102°F to 104°F); lasts 3 to 4 days
Headache	Rare	Yes
Body aches and pains	Slight	Often severe
Fatigue	Mild	Lasts 2 to 3 weeks
Extreme exhaustion	No	Early in illness; lasts a few days
Stuffy or runny nose	Yes	Occasionally
Sneezing	Yes	Occasionally
Sore throat	Yes	Occasionally
Chest discomfort and/or cough	Mild to moderate; hacking cough	Yes; may be severe
Complications	Sinus congestion, ear pain	Bronchitis, pneumonia

Sexually Transmitted Diseases

Disease	Clinical Presentation	Complications and Long-Term Risks
AIDS/HIV	May remain asymptomatic for many years Developing signs and symptoms include fatigue, fever, poor appetite, unexplained weight loss, generalized lymphadenopathy, persistent diarrhea, night sweats	Disease progression (from HIV to AIDS) is variable from a few months to 12 years. Early intervention is essential in preserving and maintaining optimal health status.
Chancroid	Painful genital ulceration(s) with tender inguinal adenopathy Ulcers may be necrotic or erosive	Chancroid has been associated with increased risk of acquiring HIV infection. Patients should be tested for other infections that cause ulcers (i.e., syphilis).
Chlamydial Cervicitis	Yellow mucopurulent cervical exudate May or may not be symptomatic Male sexual partner will likely have nongonococcal urethritis	Untreated, may develop endometritis, salpingitis, ectopic pregnancy, and/or subsequent infertility. High prevalence of coinfection with gonococcal infection. Infection during pregnancy may lead to premature rupture of membranes, pneumonia, or conjunctivitis in the infant.
Enteric Infections	Sexually transmissible enteric infections, particularly among homosexual males Abdominal pain, fever, diarrhea, vomiting	Occurs frequently with oral-genital and oral-anal contact. Infections can be life threatening if they become systemic. Organisms may be shigella, hepatitis A, giardia.
Epididymitis	May or may not be transmitted sexually Can be asymptomatic Non-sexually transmitted, is associated with a urinary tract infection Unilateral testicular pain, swelling	Usually caused by gonorrhea or chlamydia. May be caused by *Escherichia coli* after anal intercourse. Must rule out a testicular torsion before making the diagnosis of epididymitis.
Genital Warts	Soft, fleshy, painless growth(s) around the anus, penis, vulvovaginal area, cervix, urethra, or perineum	Caused by the human papillomavirus. Must rule out other causes of lesion(s) such as syphilis, etc. Lesions may cause tissue destruction. Cervical warts are associated with neoplasia.
Gonorrhea	Males may have dysuria, urinary frequency, thin clear or yellow urethral discharge	Untreated, risk of arthritis, dermatitis, bacteremia, meningitis, endocarditis. At risk: Males: epididymitis,

(*continued*)

Sexually Transmitted Diseases

Disease	Clinical Presentation	Complications and Long-Term Risks
Gonorrhea (*cont'd*)	Females may have mucopurulent vaginal discharge, abnormal menses, dysuria, or no symptoms	infertility, urethral stricture, and sterility. Females: pelvic inflammatory disease. Newborns: ophthalmia neonatorum, pneumonia
Hepatitis B	Anorexia, malaise, nausea, vomiting, abdominal pain, jaundice, skin rash, arthralgias, arthritis	Chronic hepatitis, cirrhosis, liver cancer, liver failure, death. Chronic carrier occurs in 6% to 10% of cases. Infants born with hepatitis B are at high risk for developing chronic liver disease.
Herpes genitalis (Herpes simplex type 2)	Clustered vesicles that rupture, leaving painful, shallow genital ulcer(s) that eventually crust Initial outbreak last for 14 to 21 days; subsequent outbreaks are less severe and last 8 to 12 days	Other causes of genital ulcers (syphilis, chancroid, etc.) must be ruled out.
Nongonococcal Urethritis	Dysuria, urinary frequency, mucoid to purulent urethral discharge Some men may be asymptomatic Female sexual partners may have cervicitis or PID	Can be caused by chlamydia, mycoplasma, trichomonas, or herpes simplex. Can cause urethral strictures, prostatitis, epididymitis.
Pelvic Inflammatory Disease	Lower abdominal pain, fever, cervical motion tenderness, dyspareunia, purulent vaginal discharge, dysuria, increased abdominal pain while walking.	Must rule out appendicitis or ectopic pregnancy. Risk for pelvic abscess, future ectopic pregnancy, infertility, pelvic adhesions.
Proctitis	Sexually transmitted gastrointestinal illnesses Proctitis occurs with anal intercourse, resulting in inflammation of the rectum with anorectal pain, tenesmus, and rectal discharge	May be caused by chlamydia, gonorrhea, herpes simplex, and syphilis. Among patients coinfected with HIV, herpes proctitis may be severe.
Proctocolitis	Sexually transmitted gastrointestinal illnesses Proctocolitis occurs with either anal intercourse or with oral-fecal contact, resulting in symptoms of proctitis as well as diarrhea, abdominal cramps, and inflammation of the colonic mucosa	May be caused by campylobacter, shigella, or chlamydia. Other opportunistic infections may be involved among immunosuppressed HIV patients.

(*continued*)

Sexually Transmitted Diseases

Disease	Clinical Presentation	Complications and Long-Term Risks
Pubic Lice	Slight discomfort to intense itching May have pruritic, erythematous macules, papules, or secondary excoriation in the genital area If lice are found on the eyelashes, they are usually pubic lice	Sexual partners within the last month should be treated. May develop lymphadenitis or a secondary bacterial infection of the skin or hair follicle.
Scabies	The mite burrows under the skin of the fingers, penis, and wrists Scabies among adults may be sexually transmitted, while usually *not* sexually transmitted among children Itching (worse at night), papular eruptions, and excoriation of the skin	Sexual partners, household members, and close contacts within the past month should be examined and treated. May develop a secondary infection, often with nephrotogenic streptococci.
Syphilis **Primary syphilis**	Painless, indurated ulcer (chancre) at site of infection approximately 10 days to 3 months after exposure	All genital ulcers should be suspected to be syphilitic. Patients should be tested for HIV and retested in 3 months. At-risk sex partners are those within the past 3 months plus duration of symptoms for primary syphilis, and 6 months plus duration of symptoms for secondary syphilis.
Secondary syphilis	Rash, mucocutaneous lesions, lymphadenopathy, condylomata lata Symptoms occur 4 to 6 weeks after exposure and resolve spontaneously within weeks to 12 months	
Latent syphilis	Seroreactive yet asymptomatic Can be clinically latent for a period of weeks to years Latency sometimes lasts a lifetime	Should be clinically evaluated for tertiary disease (i.e., aortitis, neurosyphilis, etc). At-risk sex partners are those within the past year for early latent syphilis.
Tertiary/late syphilis	May have cardiac, neurologic, ophthalmic, auditory, or gummatous lesions	
Neurosyphilis	May see a variety of neurologic signs and symptoms, including ataxia, bladder problems, confusion, meningitis, uveitis May be asymptomatic	Diagnosis made based on a variety of tests including: reactive serologic test results, cerebrospinal fluid (CSF) protein or cell count abnormalities, positive VDRL on CSF.
Congenital syphilis	Needs to be ruled out for infants born to mothers with untreated syphilis, mothers who received incomplete treatment, or insufficient follow-up of reported treated syphilis	Syphilis frequently causes abortion, stillbirth, and complications of prematurity of infant. Treated infants must be followed very closely and retested every 2 to 3 months. Most

(continued)

Sexually Transmitted Diseases

Disease	Clinical Presentation	Complications and Long-Term Risks
	Serologic tests for mother and infant can be negative at delivery if mother was infected late in pregnancy	infants are nonreactive by 6 months. Infants with positive CSF should be retested every 6 months and be retreated if still abnormal at 2 years.
Trichomoniasis (Vaginitis)	Profuse, thin, foamy, greenish-yellow discharge with foul odor May be asymptomatic Male partners may have urethritis	Trichomoniasis often coexists with gonorrhea. Perform a complete STD assessment if trichomoniasis is diagnosed.

Source: Grossman, V. A. (2003). *Quick Reference to Triage* (2nd ed.). Philadelphia: Lippincott Williams & Wilkins.

Triage Skills Assessment

	Time:			Time:		
	Yes	No	N/A	Yes	No	N/A

GREETING
- Greets patient courteously
- Utilizes proper opening script (identifies self)
- Gathers appropriate demographic data
- Comments:

ASSESSMENT
- Identifies emergency signs and symptoms
- Measures vital signs
- Gathers appropriate patient history
- Upgrades patient to higher level of urgency as needed (child, confused adult, foreign-language speaker)
- Makes assignment for care and acuity within appropriate time frame
- Identifies and documents patient medications and allergies
- Orders appropriate medication or diagnostic studies, per facility protocol
- Offers and documents interim care measures if not emergent (splint, ice pack, emesis basin)

(*continued*)

	Time:			Time:		
	Yes	No	N/A	Yes	No	N/A

- Documents appropriately, including assessment, nursing interventions, acuity, and disposition
- Comments:

COMMUNICATION SKILLS
- Conveys a positive image of organization
- Maintains a courteous, calm, professional demeanor
- Exhibits ability to adapt to different personalities and emotions
- Assumes control of the interview: listens attentively, interjects appropriately, and elicits necessary information
- Takes time with the patient when appropriate; efficient without compromising quality
- Uses simple, direct language that the patient understands
- Does not interrupt
- Speaks at a moderate rate with expressive modulation of tone
- Comments:

CLOSING
- Ends interview efficiently
- Informs patient of next step and expected wait
- If patient has to wait, instructs patient /family member to inform triage nurse of any changes or worsening of the problem while waiting
- Comments:

RN Name: **Reviewer:**   **Date:**

Training Exercises

IDENTIFYING APPROPRIATE NURSING INTERVENTIONS AT TRIAGE

- Select 10 different protocols that would require nursing interventions at triage based on your facility's guidelines and procedures.
- Indicate, in the space provided, the name of the protocol, page number, intervention(s), expected outcome and name of facility guideline.

Example:
Protocol: Chest Pain
Page Number _____
Intervention(s): Vital Signs, Pulse Oximetry, IV, EKG, Oxygen, Monitor, Low -Dose Aspirin, Notify Physician
Expected Outcome: Reduce discomfort, reduce damage to heart, rapidly identify potential lethal conditions, reduce time to reperfusion.
Facility Guideline: Nursing Standing Orders

1. **Protocol:** _____
   Page Number _____
   Intervention(s):
   _____

   Expected Outcome:
   _____

   Name of Facility Guideline:
   _____

2. **Protocol:** _____
   Page Number _____
   Intervention(s):
   _____

   Expected Outcome:
   _____

   Name of Facility Guideline:
   _____

3. **Protocol:** _____
   Page Number _____
   Intervention(s):
   _____

   Expected Outcome:
   _____

   Name of Facility Guideline:
   _____

4. **Protocol:** _____
   Page Number _____
   Intervention(s):
   _____

   Expected Outcome:
   _____

   Name of Facility Guideline:
   _____

5. **Protocol:** _____
   Page Number _____
   Intervention(s):
   _____

   Expected Outcome:
   _____

   Name of Facility Guideline:
   _____

(continued)

6. Protocol: _____
   Page Number _____
   Intervention(s):

   _____

   Expected Outcome:

   _____

   Name of Facility Guideline:

   _____

7. Protocol: _____
   Page Number _____
   Intervention(s):

   _____

   Expected Outcome:

   _____

   Name of Facility Guideline:

   _____

8. Protocol: _____
   Page Number _____
   Intervention(s):

   _____

   Expected Outcome:

   _____

   Name of Facility Guideline:

   _____

9. Protocol: _____
   Page Number _____
   Intervention(s):

   _____

   Expected Outcome:

   _____

   Name of Facility Guideline:

   _____

10. Protocol: _____
    Page Number _____
    Intervention(s):

    _____

    Expected Outcome:

    _____

    Name of Facility Guideline:

    _____

Name _____ Date Completed_____

Reviewed by_____ Date Reviewed_____

IDENTIFYING HOW AGE AND CHRONIC ILLNESS IMPACT THE ASSIGNMENT OF AN ACUITY LEVEL AND RISK FOR WAITING TO BE SEEN

- Select 10 different protocols that impact the acuity level based on age, medical condition, or chronic illness.
- Indicate, in the space provided, the name of the protocol, page number, condition that impacted the acuity level, acuity level, risk for waiting, nursing considerations for referral to treatment.
- Consider facility guidelines for appropriate waiting times for each category.

Example:
Protocol: Chest Pain
Page Number _____
Condition Impacting Acuity: Age >35 yr and heart palpitations; recent trauma, childbirth, surgery, or history of blood clotting problems; history of diabetes; congestive heart failure or blood clotting problems
Acuity Level: Level 2
Risk for Waiting: High risk
Nursing Considerations: Emergent, Refer for treatment within minutes

1. Protocol: _____
   Page Number _____
   Condition Impacting Acuity:

   _____

   Acuity Level: _____
   Risk for Waiting:_____
   Nursing Consideration:

   _____

2. **Protocol:** _____
   Page Number _____
   Condition Impacting Acuity:

   _____

   Acuity Level: _____
   Risk for Waiting:_____
   Nursing Consideration:

   _____

3. **Protocol:** _____
   Page Number _____
   Condition Impacting Acuity:

   _____

   Acuity Level: _____
   Risk for Waiting:_____
   Nursing Consideration:

   _____

4. **Protocol:** _____
   Page Number _____
   Condition Impacting Acuity:

   _____

   Acuity Level: _____
   Risk for Waiting:_____
   Nursing Consideration:

   _____

5. **Protocol:** _____
   Page Number _____
   Condition Impacting Acuity:

   _____

   Acuity Level: _____
   Risk for Waiting:_____
   Nursing Consideration:

   _____

6. **Protocol:** _____
   Page Number _____
   Condition Impacting Acuity:

   _____

   Acuity Level: _____
   Risk for Waiting:_____
   Nursing Consideration:

   _____

7. **Protocol:** _____
   Page Number _____
   Condition Impacting Acuity:

   _____

   Acuity Level: _____
   Risk for Waiting:_____
   Nursing Consideration:

   _____

8. **Protocol:** _____
   Page Number _____
   Condition Impacting Acuity:

   _____

   Acuity Level: _____
   Risk for Waiting:_____
   Nursing Consideration:

   _____

9. **Protocol:** _____
   Page Number _____
   Condition Impacting Acuity:

   _____

   Acuity Level: _____
   Risk for Waiting:_____
   Nursing Consideration:

   _____

10. **Protocol:** _____
    Page Number _____
    Condition Impacting Acuity:

    _____

    Acuity Level: _____
    Risk for Waiting:_____
    Nursing Consideration:

    _____

Name _____ Date Completed_____

Reviewed by_____ Date Reviewed_____

(continued)

SCENARIO PRACTICE

The purpose of this exercise is to help the nurse orient to the triage protocols and teach new nurses to recognize an emergent situation, appropriate disposition, and what to anticipate in terms of utilization of resources. In addition, it can assist the nurse in identifying when it is appropriate to initiate diagnostic studies and interventions based on facility guidelines.

For each scenario described below, identify in the space provided:
- The acuity level and triage category based on the 5-tier triage system
- Time frame to be seen by the physician (consider facility policy for semi-urgent and non-urgent patients)
- Anticipated nursing considerations, interventions, medical diagnostics, procedures, and consultations
- The protocol used and associated page number

EXAMPLE: A 58-year-old male has a chief complaint of midsternal chest pain, nausea, and diaphoresis for the past 2 hours. He describes his pain as 8/10 on the pain scale. His vital signs are BP 140/90, P 96, R 22.

Acuity Level: 2 High Risk **Triage Category**: Emergent
Time Frame to Be Seen: Should not wait to be seen
Nursing Considerations: Anticipate IV, labs, EKG, monitor, medications, O_2
Protocol Referenced: Chest pain **Page Number** _____

1. A 26-year-old female has a chief complaint of urinary frequency and burning when she urinates. She denies flank pain or vaginal discharge. Her last menstrual period was 2 weeks ago. She is taking birth-control pills. Her vital signs are BP 118/72, P 70, R 18, T 97.6°F.

   Acuity Level: _____ Triage Category: _____
   Time Frame to Be Seen: _____
   Nursing Considerations: _____
   Protocol Referenced: _____ Page Number _____

2. A 17-year-old male has a chief complaint of a sore throat since yesterday. He denies swollen or tender nodes or exudate in the back of the throat. He is able to swallow and handle his secretions well and speak in full sentences. He describes his pain as a 5/10 on the pain scale. His vital signs are BP 114/76, P 70, R 18, T 98.6°F.

   Acuity Level: _____ Triage Category: _____
   Time Frame to Be Seen: _____
   Nursing Considerations: _____
   Protocol Referenced: _____ Page Number _____

3. A 19-year-old male has a chief complaint of nausea since this morning. He states he "threw up" once this morning. He denies diarrhea or abdominal pain. He has been able to tolerate fluids. His vital signs are BP 120/76, P 80, R 18, T 98.4°F.

   Acuity Level: _____ Triage Category: _____
   Time Frame to Be Seen: _____
   Nursing Considerations: _____
   Protocol Referenced:_____ Page Number _____

4. A 42-year-old female has a chief complaint of a severe headache, described as the "worst headache of my life," that started 1 hour prior to arrival. She describes her pain as 10/10 on the pain scale. She is awake and alert but obviously uncomfortable. She denies a head injury or history of headaches. Her vital signs are BP 150/80, P 90, R 20, T 98.2°F.

   Acuity Level: _____ Triage Category: _____
   Time Frame to Be Seen: _____
   Nursing Considerations: _____
   Protocol Referenced: _____ Page Number _____

5. A 68-year-old male reportedly collapsed at the mall and has been brought in by the paramedics. His wife states that he had been complaining about chest discomfort before collapsing. He was defibrillated 3 times and CPR has been in progress for the past 20 minutes. His pupils remain reactive to light.

Acuity Level: _____ Triage Category: _____

Time Frame to Be Seen: _____

Nursing Considerations: _____

Protocol Referenced: _____ Page Number _____

6. A 24-year-old male injured his ankle while playing basketball 2 hours ago. He reportedly came down on his ankle and felt a pop. The ankle is now painful, swollen, and ecchymotic. He states that he is unable to bear weight on that extremity due to the discomfort. He describes the pain as 6/10 on the pain scale. His vital signs are BP 110/60, P 80, R 20, T 98.2°F.

Acuity Level: _____ Triage Category: _____

Time Frame to Be Seen: _____

Nursing Considerations: _____

Protocol Referenced: _____ Page Number _____

7. A 24-year-old female has a chief complaint of dizziness and states her mind "feels fuzzy, she can't think straight." She states she has a history of diabetes and took her insulin this morning but can't remember whether or not she ate breakfast. Her vital signs are BP 118/70, P 70, R 16, T 98.2°F.

Acuity Level: _____ Triage Category: _____

Time Frame to Be Seen: _____

Nursing Considerations: _____

Protocol Referenced: _____ Page Number _____

8. An 82-year-old female has a chief complaint of "weakness, a little confused and has no appetite." Her daughter states that she has generally been healthy and active up until the past few days. She also states that her mother had been complaining of "some burning with urination." Her vital signs are BP 118/70, P 80, R 18, T 100.6°F.

Acuity Level: _____ Triage Category: _____

Time Frame to Be Seen: _____

Nursing Considerations: _____

Protocol Referenced: _____ Page Number _____

9. A 19-year-old male has a chief complaint that he was stabbed in the chest twice by his girlfriend about 30 minutes ago. He states he is having some difficulty catching his breath. He is pale and his vital signs are BP 70/40, P 128, R 26, T 98.1°F.

Acuity Level: _____ Triage Category: _____

Time Frame to Be Seen: _____

Nursing Considerations: _____

Protocol Referenced: _____ Page Number _____

10. A 67-year-old male has a chief complaint of sudden weakness on his left side. He has a noticeable facial droop and is unsteady on his feet. He states that the symptoms started about 1 hour prior to arrival. His vital signs are BP 160/94, P 98, R 20, T 100.1°F.

Acuity Level: _____ Triage Category: _____

Time Frame to Be Seen: _____

Nursing Considerations: _____

Protocol Referenced:_____ Page Number _____

11. A 17-year-old male has a chief complaint of left ear pain since last night. He states this happens every time he goes swimming, but this time he can't seem to shake it. His vital signs are BP 116/72, P 74, R 16, T 98.2°F.

Acuity Level: _____ Triage Category: _____

Time Frame to Be Seen: _____

Nursing Considerations: _____

Protocol Referenced: _____ Page Number _____

12. A 33-year-old male has a chief complaint of nausea, vomiting, and diarrhea for 3 days. He states that he has been ill since returning from a camping trip a few days ago. He has been unable to keep anything down and nothing has worked to stop the vomiting or diarrhea. His vital signs are BP 106/62, P 88, R 18, T 98.4°F.

Acuity Level: _____ Triage Category: _____

Time Frame to Be Seen: _____

(continued)

Nursing Considerations: _____

Protocol Referenced: _____ Page Number ____

13. A 72-year-old male has a chief complaint of abdominal pain. He states it is "pretty bad" and radiates into his back. His wife states that the pain started about 2 hours ago and he nearly fainted several times prior to arrival in the Emergency Department. His vital signs are BP 174/92, P 88, R 20, T 98.2°F, Pain Scale 7/10.

Acuity Level: _____ Triage Category: _____

Time Frame to Be Seen: _____

Nursing Considerations: _____

Protocol Referenced: _____ Page Number ____

14. A 42-year-old male is concerned he may have an allergic reaction to something he ate. He recently ingested some peanut oil by accident and states he has had a severe allergy to peanuts in the past. His vital signs are BP 144/88, P 108, R 24, T 98.2°F. He suddenly collapses after you take his vital signs.

Acuity Level: _____ Triage Category: _____

Time Frame to Be Seen: _____

Nursing Considerations: _____

Protocol Referenced: _____ Page Number ____

15. A 48-year-old male has a chief complaint of vomiting blood and abdominal pain. He is pale and diaphoretic. His vital signs are BP 80/50, P 118, R 24, T 98.2°F. Pain scale 6/10.

Acuity Level: _____ Triage Category: _____

Time Frame to Be Seen: _____

Nursing Considerations: _____

Protocol Referenced: _____ Page Number ____

16. A 17-year-old female has a chief complaint of dental pain. She has a history of right upper molar pain and swelling for the past 10 days. She states she has been unable to get in to see a dentist for the past 2 weeks. She is alert, oriented,

and breathing without difficulty. Her vital signs are BP 126/70, P 68, R 18, T 98.4°F. Pain scale 6/10.

Acuity Level: _____ Triage Category: _____

Time Frame to Be Seen: _____

Nursing Considerations: _____

Protocol Referenced: _____ Page Number ____

17. A 28-year-old female has a chief complaint of a headache, rated 7/10 on the pain scale. She has nausea and photophobia and states this episode is similar to other migraines she has experienced in the past but this one has not responded to her usual homecare measures and pain medications. Her vital signs are BP 118/68, P 88, R 22, T 98.2°F.

Acuity Level: _____ Triage Category: _____

Time Frame to Be Seen: _____

Nursing Considerations: _____

Protocol Referenced: _____ Page Number ____

18. A 34-year-old female has a chief complaint of facial injuries, including ecchymosis to both eyes, a swollen lip, and dried blood around the nose. She states a book fell off the shelf and hit her in the face. Her vital signs are BP 138/78, P 88, R 22, T 98.2°F. Pain scale 5/10.

Acuity Level: _____ Triage Category: _____

Time Frame to Be Seen: _____

Nursing Considerations: _____

Protocol Referenced: _____ Page Number ____

19. A 77-year-old female has a chief complaint of a shoulder injury. She states she tripped and fell about 3 hours ago on her right shoulder. She is able to ambulate and has pain and swelling to the right upper arm. She has limited range of motion in the right arm. Her circulation, sensation, and movement are intact. Her vital signs are BP 138/78, P 88, R 20, T 98.2°F. Pain scale 7/10.

Acuity Level: _____ Triage Category: _____

Time Frame to Be Seen: _____

Nursing Considerations: _____

Protocol Referenced: _____ Page Number _____

20. A 28-year-old male has a chief complaint of splashing cleaning fluid in both eyes 20 minutes ago. He tried to splash cold water into his eyes immediately afterward. His eyes are reddened, swollen, and painful. He rates his pain a 7/10 on the pain scale. His vital signs are BP 128/78, P 88, R 20, T 98.2°F.

Acuity Level: _____ Triage Category: _____

Time Frame to Be Seen: _____

Nursing Considerations: _____

Protocol Referenced: _____ Page Number _____

Index